Mutagenesis in Sub-Mammalian Systems

Mutagenesis in Sub-Mammalian Systems
status and significance

Edited by G. E. Paget

Director, Inveresk Research International

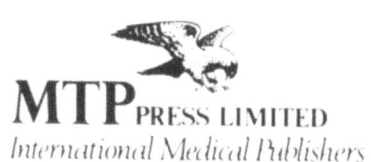

MTP PRESS LIMITED
International Medical Publishers

Published by

MTP Press Limited
Falcon House
Cable Street
Lancaster
England

ISBN-13: 978-94-011-6641-6   e-ISBN-13: 978-94-011-6639-3
DOI: 10.1007/978-94-011-6639-3

Contents

Mutagenesis in Sub-Mammalian Systems *was sponsored
and organized by Inveresk Research International. The
meeting was the third in their series "Topics in Toxicology"
aimed at producing meetings on subjects of topical importance to toxicologists.*

List of Contributors

Professor B. N. AMES
Biochemistry Department, University of California,
Berkeley, California, USA

D. ANDERSON
Central Toxicology Laboratory, Imperial Chemical Industries Ltd,
Alderley Park, Macclesfield, Cheshire

J. ASHBY
Central Toxicology Laboratory, Imperial Chemical Industries Ltd,
Alderley Park, Macclesfield, Cheshire

Professor (Emeritus) C. AUERBACH
31 Upper Gray Street, Edinburgh 9

Professor B. A. BRIDGES
MRC Cell Mutation Unit, University of Sussex,
Falmer, Brighton, Sussex

B. J. DEAN
Shell Research Ltd, Tunstall Laboratory,
Sittingbourne, Kent

M. H. DRAPER
Department of Health & Social Security, Alexander Fleming House,
Elephant & Castle, London SE1 6BY

Professor L. EHRENBERG
Stockholm University, Wallenberglaboratoriet, Lilla Frescati,
S-104 05 Stockholm 50, Sweden

D. B. McGREGOR
Inveresk Research International, Inveresk Gate,
Musselburgh, Midlothian

P. OFTEDAL
Institute of General Genetics, University of Oslo,
PO Boks 1031, Blindern, Oslo 3, Norway

J. A. STYLES
Central Toxicology Laboratory, Imperial Chemical Industries Ltd,
Alderley Park, Macclesfield, Cheshire

Series Preface
Topics in Toxicology

Toxicology is a science that stands at the intersection of several interests and disciplines. These intersecting forces are by no means all scientific since some are legal and some are commercial. All have valid things to say about the conduct and interpretation of toxicity experiments. The practising toxicologist must bear all these sometimes conflicting forces in mind as he carries out his duties. This is especially true, of course, of the toxicologist in industry.

Toxicology is also a field in which contract research particularly flourishes and a number of major contract research companies have established over the years a reputation for contributing usefully to the practice of this skill. These contract research organisations are particularly favoured to develop an appreciation of the problems of the industrial toxicologist, since it is very common for such a company to service the toxicological needs of companies in several sectors of industry producing new chemical compounds, and the contract research company, therefore, is aware of a wider diversity of problems than probably affects a single toxicologist in one industry.

Among the problems of which all toxicologists in industry are aware and particularly so those in contract research companies, is the relative paucity of fora for adequate toxicological discussion. There are, it is true, at least two major societies concerned with problems of toxicology, the European Society of Toxicology and the Society of Toxicology in America. Although performing a useful function, these societies are now so large, and cater for such a wide spread of interests and contain so many individuals whose interests in toxicology is at most peripheral, that many toxicologists feel they do not provide an adequate platform for discussion of the most immediate and important issues affecting toxicology at any one time. The very size and complexity of these societies means that the organization of their meetings and the topics for their symposia must be chosen many months, and indeed years, in advance. Thus issues of current importance cannot usually be dealt with while they are still alive.

Inveresk Research International, a contract research company operating, among other areas of contract research, in the general field of toxicology, feels that there is a need for small, highly specialized and specific, meetings, arranged at relatively short notice to cover important current issues in toxicology and has instituted the series 'Topics in Toxicology' to meet this need. The subjects for these meetings are, as far as possible, ones of immediate concern to practising toxicologists in industry. They bring together, as far as possible, the most authoritative opinions bearing on the particular subject. Subjects chosen within the general constraint of current interest, ones which stand at the intersection of at least two of the several strands of interest that control industrial toxicology.

G. E. Paget

Foreword

In the past few years there has been a steadily increasing awareness among the scientific community generally, and toxicologists particularly, of several important and related facts and propositions. In the first place it has been thought for many years that a high proportion of human cancers may have environmental causes – this probability arises from the widely differing cancer rates for various geographical locations. Second, it is evident that a very large number – perhaps of the order of 10^5 – of chemical compounds for all sorts of uses has been introduced into the human environment, and that a relatively small proportion of them – perhaps of the order of 10^3 – have been tested at all for safety and even fewer have been tested in a way that could be regarded as completely adequate. Finally it is clear that the physical, technical and financial resources required to test the untested 99 % adequately in a reasonable length of time simply do not exist, and are unlikely to exist for a very long time to come if they ever do.

This complex of facts has caused an intense search for short-term methods for predicting carcinogenicity with some degree of reliability sufficient at the very least to set priorities for longer-term testing, or, as Ames argues persuasively, for decisive actions. It is relevant in this connection that for many years one of the mechanisms proposed for the pathogenesis of cancer is the development of a somatic mutation, that is a change in the DNA of a somatic cell, which allows the development of the highly abnormal clone of cells that constitute a cancer. From this it is but a short step to the development of a number of methods, and pre-eminently of a series of bacterial test systems by Ames, to detect mutations in simple systems in which the results can be obtained in days or weeks rather than years and at a cost of hundreds rather than hundreds of thousands of pounds, and which it is hoped will predict both the carcinogenic and the genetic hazards of human exposure.

The growth of such systems and their widespread use has been pheno-menal. In 1973 IRI was one of the first commercial laboratories in the world to establish a department in the charge of a distinguished research scientist with the sole purpose of developing methods for the study of mutagens. For 2 years not a single contract for such work was placed by any industrial client. Now the laboratory is growing at a considerable rate because of the demand for its skills, and a great number of major chemical manufacturers have established groups of their own – ICI Ltd. and Shell Ltd. merit special mention for the brilliance and commitment of their work in this field.

Such work, of course, can only adequately be done by those skilled in the rapidly advancing science of genetic toxicology. The basic knowledge, indeed even the jargon, lies outside the experience of most toxicologists and research managers, yet it is they who must make, or recommend to wholly non-scientific management, decisions often of great moment based upon the work of the specialist geneticists. In a field advancing as rapidly as is that of mutagenic studies currently, it is difficult as a non-specialist to evaluate the sometimes conflicting claims and techniques of different groups, while the specialist is often an enthusiast utterly persuaded of the significant importance of his own work.

To shed some light in this area of debate, IRI established its third discussion in the series of 'Topics in Toxicology'. The various distinguished contributors were asked to address themselves primarily to the non-specialist but informed scientist, and to endeavour to lay out for him the present state of methods, and even more of interpretation in this field. The result was highly satisfactory to all who attended the meeting and even in publication the quite unique flavour of scientific presentations of great profundity and clarity comes over. None of the contributors has pulled any punches in presenting the technical facts, but the conscientious reader will be left with a clear impression of a developing field of study that will with some certainty serve as a basis for useful decision and action in years to come, and will become acquainted with the factual basis, and the interpretative insights of this fascinating field of study that we must learn to call 'genetic toxicology'.

G. E. Paget

Introduction
Lord Ritchie-Calder

It is sheer effrontery for me to be standing in front of you as your Conference Chairman, but I was quite immodestly flattered by the invitation. I may have one supreme qualification for this task – I am prepared to take on the odium and the responsibility for making sure that speakers keep to their times.

If I had to establish my own credentials for being here, I would claim to be an expert on experts, as my one expertise is experts. As a science writer I have learned to get behind the disembodied papers in scientific journals, to get at the people actually on the job, to find out what they are doing, how they are doing it, and what makes them tick. As an expert on experts I am enormously impressed by the array of experts assembled here, demonstrating concern with a topic which is surely – surely – one of the most important in the world today. The implications of the topic certainly are.

On the subject matter, as a science writer I can claim to have been the first to introduce DNA to the general public. As Science Editor of the *News Chronicle* I had hammered out an article with Watson and Crick, and with Maurice Wilkins and Rosa Franklin – who should have had that posthumous Nobel Prize – and we had made DNA intelligible to the newspaper reader. I started that article with 'Deoxyribonucleic acid – deoxyribonucleic acid – deoxyribonucleic acid – repeat it, spell it, remember it. It is perhaps the most portentous term you will ever learn . . .'. And I still believe so.

Remember what we did with the secret of matter. We exploded it as a cataclysm of atomic fire. I put it to you, what will we do with the secret of life if we are as irresponsible in our handling of it ?

In the discussions at this Symposium we shall be getting down to the very heart of the scientific ethic. Over a century ago, Claude Bernard, the famous French physiologist, said:

. . . science teaches us to doubt, and in ignorance to refrain.

He was not implying a moratorium on science. On the contrary, he was insisting that we proceed from one toehold of knowledge to the next. It is like venturing into an uncharted minefield of ignorance with a mine detector. The job of science is to perfect those detectors.

Over 40 years ago when vitamins were the 'in' thing and becoming a popular cult, the scientist who had received the Nobel Prize for his work on vitamins, Sir Frederick Gowland Hopkins, said to me:

All that I have learned about vitamins has taught me what I do not know about vitamins. A vitamin is a unit by which we measure our ignorance. Every food factor which is discovered is a reminder of the factors we have not discovered.

How much more so is that true in the case of the mutagens.

In the case of Hopkins, that was the true humility of science, in contrast with what he himself described as 'the lusty self-confidence of Liebig in the nineteenth century'.

Looking through the scope of the proceedings here, and through the papers, I am impressed by the way in which the mine detectors are being refined, and the proper awareness of the booby traps that can trigger off mutagenesis, carcinogenesis, teratogenesis and iatrogenesis – words which in my old job as a science writer I should have had great difficulty in spelling out and defining – but I would have done it. I expect, in fact I hope, that there will be scepticism in the discussions, and I hope for contention. I am looking forward to that because that is what a scientific conference is all about.

SECTION ONE

General Background to Mutagenesis Studies

1

Mutagenesis – the significance of DNA damage for man
B. A. Bridges

It is almost exactly 25 years since the elucidation of the structure of DNA, the key molecule of all free living organisms. It is DNA which is responsible for the everyday life of living things, containing the information necessary to make the enzymes and proteins that go to make up the functioning systems within the cell. It is DNA also which is responsible for passing on from one generation to another the information necessary to generate a new individual, whether it be the simplest bacterium, or one of the various types of cell within an animal or plant, or the complete unbelievably complex organism that is man. All human attributes, from the body of a Muhammad Ali in his prime, through the creative genius of a Mozart, to the penetrating intelligence of an Einstein, derive from the information encoded in a linear sequence of purine and pyrimidine bases in DNA, and from the way in which this information is expressed and interacts with the individual's environment.

DNA is the object of study, at different levels, of both geneticists and molecular biologists and it has been obvious to these workers for many years that any interference with the DNA in a living organism may have the most profound consequences. The concern of scientists for such consequences in man has led over the last decade to the creation of a new field, genetic toxicology, in which lies the subject of this present meeting.

When the information in an organism's DNA is altered in some way, its descendants may show altered characteristics. Such a heritable change is known as a mutation. In one sense there is no such thing as an organism without mutations; we all contain slightly different packages of genes (as the bits of information in DNA are called). Nevertheless most of the slight differences between our DNAs are compatible with a healthy life and the gene packages that have evolved are so finely tuned that most further mutations are likely to be deleterious. Harmful mutations are indeed present in the human population to a far greater extent than is commonly realized, but before discussing these it is necessary to consider the implications of diploidy.

Diploidy is the state whereby the fertilized egg (and most of the cells derived from it) contains two complete sets of information, one from the sperm (paternal genes) and one from the egg (maternal genes). Some mutations can express themselves even in the presence of a 'normal' or wild-type copy of the same gene and are called *dominant*. Others, called *recessive*, are expressed only in the absence of a wild-type gene. A recessive mutation inherited, say, from the father will only be seen when it is partnered by a similar mutation in the DNA inherited from the mother (a situation described as *homozygous*). (Of course there is a whole range of intermediate conditions between dominant and recessive which complicates matters to some extent.) There is an exception, in that all mutations present on the X and Y chromosomes, whether dominant or recessive, are expressed in males since the latter contain only one copy of the genes in these chromosomes. Such mutations are termed sex-linked and are almost always on the X chromosome, the Y being relatively inactive.

GENETIC DISEASE IN MAN

Individual mutations in man sufficiently harmful to show up as severe disease conditions are relatively rare yet collectively they add up to a very significant health burden, bearing in mind that those afflicted often require medical attention for the whole of their lives. Table 1.1 lists the major dominant and sex-linked diseases due to gene mutations which together may account for more than 1 in every 400 live births. If one includes less serious conditions the figure could be as much as 1 in every 100 births. These categories are important because the frequencies reflect current

Table 1.1   Some of the commoner autosomal dominant (A) and sex-linked (B) diseases (total frequencies around 2 and 0.8 per 1000 live births respectively)

A	B
Huntington's chorea	Duchene muscular dystrophy
Neurofibromatosis	Becker muscular dystrophy
Mytotonia dystrophica	Haemophilia A
Epiloia	Haemophilia B
Multiple intestinal polyposis	Ichthyosis
Gardner's syndrome	Severe mental retardation
Bilateral polycystic disease of the kidney	Severe childhood deafness
(adult form)	Childhood blindness
Achondroplasia	Testicular feminization
Diaphyseal aclasis (multiple exostoses)	
Marfan's syndrome	
Childhood blindness	
Retinoblastoma	
Severe childhood deafness	
Hereditary spherocytosis	
Cleft lip and/or palate with lip pits	
Acute intermittent porphyria	
Porphyria variegata	

Table 1.2   Some of the commoner autosomal recessive diseases (total frequency around 2.4 per 1000 live births)

Severe mental retardation	Phenylketonuria
Severe childhood deafness	Other aminoacidurias
Childhood blindness	Galactosaemia
Cystic fibrosis	Mucopolysaccharidoses
Adrenogenital syndromes	Tay–Sachs disease
Oculocutaneous albinism	Acute spinal muscular atrophy

mutation rates in the human population. This is not true for the recessive diseases (Table 1.2) many of which are maintained in the population by selection in the heterozygous state.

Among the commonest genetic disorders are those which involve sufficiently gross alterations of the genetic material that they can be discerned microscopically. Down's syndrome (mongolism), for example, affects around 1 in 200 live births. These chromosome abnormalities affect a total of nearly 1 in 100 live births.

The chromosomal and defined single gene diseases altogether amount to as much as 1 in 80 live births, but in addition to these there are the congenital malformations (of which perhaps half are genetic) and complex disorders (of which the genetic contribution is perhaps one-third). These

may raise the total overt genetic contribution to human disease to around
1 in every 25 births.

Spontaneous mutations have been shown to occur in every organism in
which they have been sought, and they may also be induced by a variety of
physical and chemical agents (mutagens) most of which have the ability to
interact with DNA in some way. There is no reason to believe that man
will be different from other organisms in being susceptible to these agents.

MUTAGENIC EFFECTS OF CHEMICALS IN MAN

Despite this substantial genetic burden that mankind carries, there is
remarkably little evidence about whether environmental factors (such as
chemical mutagens) actually do influence the levels of genetic disease in
different parts of the world or among different groups of people.

The largest group of people who are regularly exposed to significant
quantities of mutagens over long periods of time are cigarette smokers.
Cigarette smoke contains many mutagens, some of them potent, and the
urine of cigarette smokers who inhale contains readily demonstrable
mutagenic activity[1]. It is among the progeny of this group of people that
one might expect to observe additional mutations. In particular one should
look for effects among the children of men who smoke rather than women,
since in the latter case teratogenic effects on the developing foetus could
mask any genetic effect. Two effects have recently been reported[2] as
correlating with paternal cigarette smoking in a German study, namely
perinatal mortality and the incidence of major congenital abnormalities
(Table 1.3). The latter are particularly notable because of the clear relation
to the number of cigarettes smoked.

These data were thrown up by a study in which about a dozen possible
correlating factors were considered and they urgently need confirmation
in an epidemiological study specifically designed to monitor the effect of
smoking. Until such confirmation is obtained the results must be regarded

Table 1.3   Major congenital malformations (A) and perinatal mortality (B) as a function of paternal consumption
of cigarettes[2]

Cigarettes smoked daily	A	B
0	0.8%	3.0%
1–10	1.4%	2.5%
>10	2.1%	4.5%
	($p < 0.01$)	($p < 0.01$)

as preliminary. Nevertheless, it is worth while examining the implications of the result if it should turn out to be true. If the average consumption of smokers is around 10 cigarettes per day, it would not be unreasonable to take a figure of 1.8% for the incidence of major congenital abnormalities among their children compared with 0.8% among those of non-smokers. The excess of abnormalities in the whole population, if 50% of fathers smoked cigarettes, would be 0.5%. Thus almost 40% of the major congenital abnormalities in the population could be attributed to paternal smoking. That would amount to around 3000 per year in the UK. Furthermore, if about half of the congenital abnormalities were genetic in origin, this would imply that the mutation frequency as measured in the children of smokers (reflecting presumably dominant mutations) is elevated at least 2.5-fold above that measured in the children of non-smokers. The difference in mutation *rate* could be even higher because not all dominant mutations contributing to the abnormalities will be newly arising. Such an effect, if genuine, would be of great importance to the human gene pool, quite apart from adding a new dimension to the moral dilemma confronting cigarette smokers and the companies and governments which profit from their addiction. The need for new studies either to refute the German results or to establish them more securely is correspondingly great.

One of the problems in detecting genetic effects in man is that large numbers of offspring have to be monitored to accumulate usable numbers of congenital abnormalities and the majority of single gene defects (which are even rarer) are not manifest at birth. Moreover, since dominant gene mutations persist in the population for an average of around five generations only about 20% of dominant mutations will be newly arisen in any given generation. Thus the mutation *rate* would need to be elevated 5-fold to produce a doubling of the *frequency* in the first generation. Thus it is often impracticable to study for heritable mutations the relatively small groups of people who are occupationally exposed. Chromosomal damage may, however, give rise to foetal death and the incidence of spontaneous abortion has been used in several studies. In a retrospective study[3], spontaneous abortion among the wives of vinyl chloride polymerization workers was found to be significantly elevated compared to the same couples prior to the husband working with vinyl chloride or to the wives of control workers in the rubber or PVC fabrication industries (Table 1.4). As with many epidemiological investigations, criticisms have been levelled at this study[4] (and refuted[5]), but it does serve to illustrate the potentiality of the method, particularly in the field of occupational exposure.

The method has also been used in two studies on groups exposed to

Table 1.4   Age-adjusted foetal death rates per 100 pregnancies as a function of primary exposure of husband to vinyl chloride[3]

	Controls*	Primary exposure†
Before husband's exposure	6.9 (159)‡	6.1 (148)
After husband's exposure	8.8 (273)	15.8 (139)§

* Rubber and PVC fabrication workers
† Vinyl chloride polymerization workers
‡ Number of pregnancies
§ Significantly greater than control group ($p < 0.05$) and the study group before husbands' exposure ($p < 0.02$) by age-adjusted chi-square testing

anaesthetic gases. In 1974 an *ad hoc* committee of the American Society of Anaesthesiologists (ASA) reported[6] that spouses of male members of the Associations of Operating Room Nurses and of Operating Room Technicians (AORN/T) had a higher incidence of spontaneous abortions than wives of unexposed members of the American Nursing Association. The numbers, however, were small and the significance, at $p = 0.04$, was dubious. Spouses of male members of the ASA and the American Association of Nurse Anaesthetists (AANA) showed no significant increase over spouses of male members of the American Academy of Pediatrics (AAP). In the same investigation wives of members of the ASA, AANA and AORN/T had uniformly higher rates of congenital abnormalities among their live-born infants than wives of members of the AAP or ANA. In the second study on exposed and unexposed dentists[7], the rate of spontaneous abortions among wives of the former was significantly elevated ($p < 0.01$). In both these studies there were also significant effects in the offspring of exposed females but it cannot be discerned whether such effects were genetic or teratogenic.

These few examples probably comprise the entire literature on chemical induction of heritable effects in man.

CARCINOGENS AND SOMATIC MUTATION

If I have dwelt overlong on heritable effects it is because they have received little appreciation among toxicologists. In contrast the involvement of DNA-damaging agents in carcinogenesis has captured the headlines. I reviewed this field recently[8] and it forms the subject of Professor Ames's chapter later in this volume. There is therefore little need for me to discuss further the correlation between the mutagenic and carcinogenic properties of chemicals. Both are the consequences of damage to DNA. In the case of carcinogenesis there is much we still have to learn about the mechanisms involved. Certainly there are factors other than DNA-damaging agents that work to raise the level of human cancer, but there is little doubt that some of the cellular changes are a consequence of heritable alterations that can be operationally defined as somatic mutations. Although environmental factors have been held to be responsible for the great majority of human cancers[9], we still do not know the contribution that can be attributed to DNA damaging agents. Nevertheless our ability to detect DNA-damaging agents with a variety of simple test systems is proving to be a powerful tool in cancer prevention.

Geneticists are confident that exposure of human tissues to mutagenic agents must lead to a variety of mutations, apart from malignancy, in the somatic cells. From our knowledge of the importance of DNA we can be sure that a proportion of somatic mutations will be deleterious to health but at the present time such effects remain largely in the realm of speculation. Somatic mutations have long been hypothesized to be involved in part of the process of senescence. More recently atherosclerotic plaques, which kill more people than any other disease, have been shown to be largely clonal, that is derived from a single cell. This has led to the hypothesis that they are due to mutations initiated by mutagenic agents and has opened a new approach to research into the causes of vascular disease[10].

Whatever their consequences for the health of the individual may be, somatic mutations certainly occur and can be demonstrated in peripheral blood lymphocytes during short-term culture. The microscopic observation of chromosomal damage in such cells (cytogenetics) is now well established[11]. More recently a radioautographic technique has been developed for detecting 6-thioguanine-resistant variants in such cells[12]. These probably reflect gene mutations. Other techniques for observing gene mutations are under development and, together with the cytogenetic techniques, will have a large part to play in the detection of human exposure to mutagens and in the calibration of human response. Already a number of large companies are monitoring their work force cytogenetically[13].

DNA REPLICATION AND REPAIR

With a molecule of such importance as DNA it is not surprising that cells have developed a sophisticated set of devices to prevent too many errors creeping into the encoded information. Most depend upon the double-stranded nature of DNA so that two copies of the genetic information are present within the same molecule. From studies with bacteria we know that when the molecule is being replicated, there are at least four checks on the correctness of each base as it is inserted opposite the parental strand base which is its template. Firstly the ability of the new base to form a hydrogen bonded pair with the parental strand base ensures a fairly good degree of basic pairing. Secondly the polymerase molecule monitors the new base before linking it to the growing chain. Thirdly if an incorrect base has been inserted, another part of the polymerase molecule has an exonuclease function ('edit-function' or 'proof-reading') which may detect and immediately cut the bond that has just been formed thus releasing the incorrect base. Finally, should an incorrect base escape detection thus far, an endonuclease exists which can detect the mismatched base pair, cut out the wrong base and allow a polymerase to have another chance to insert a correct base.

Despite all these checks, incorrect bases do escape detection and these may result in so-called spontaneous mutations. Some chemicals may induce mutations by interfering with the fidelity of one or more of these steps of replication. Most chemical mutagens, however, are not so subtle. Rather, they cause a variety of types of chemical damage to DNA, most of which must be repaired if the DNA is to continue to function and the cell to survive.

Again, from studies with bacteria we know of at least three basic ways in which cells can repair such damage, two fundamentally accurate and one fundamentally error-prone. For a more detailed discussion of DNA repair see Lehmann and Bridges[14]. The importance of the error-prone repair mechanism, at least in bacteria, is that it is the major pathway for the production of base pair substitution mutations. Frameshift mutations, resulting from the deletion or insertion of one or two bases, arise by a different mechanism that is less well understood.

DNA repair in human cells is currently the subject of much attention and it is already clear that if the basic processes are the same as in bacteria, they are considerably more complex in their operation. In studies with bacteria, the isolation and study of mutants blocked at one or more stages of DNA repair was crucial in revealing the details of the mechanisms of both repair and mutagenesis. A similar approach, using cells from humans believed to be deficient in DNA repair, is currently a major project in our laboratory. There are now nearly two dozen genetically different diseases in man in which cultured skin cells show sensitivity to one or more DNA damaging agents. Individuals with these diseases, most of which are recessive, are of course rare. In many cases they are abnormally prone to develop malignant disease (for example xeroderma pigmentosum, Fanconi's anaemia, ataxia telangiectasia).

These repair-deficient human genes are of interest to more than molecular geneticists. Because they are recessive they are carried in the heterozygous state by a significant proportion of the 'normal' population. It has been estimated that 1% of the population carry the ataxia telangiectasia gene and 0.3% the gene for Fanconi's anaemia. The significance of this lies in the fact that relatives of patients with both these diseases have been reported to be at greater risk of developing cancer than the general population. The possibility thus arises that heterozygotes could form a significantly large high-risk group for cancer (and perhaps for mutation) within the total population. There is, of course, also the possibility of high-risk groups due to differences in metabolism of mutagens and carcinogens. If such differences are taken together with differences in DNA repair, individual susceptibility to mutagens and carcinogens could vary widely in the human population, with a group, small in proportion but not in numbers, at considerable risk. If this were so, it would have significant consequences for the way in which mutagens and carcinogens are regulated and controlled. Hereditary conditions in man attributed to deficiencies in DNA repair have been recently reviewed by Arlett and Lehmann[15].

CONCLUSION

Of course, genetic toxicology is not the entire field of toxicology; nevertheless I hope that I have succeeded in giving an impression of the importance of DNA and of the consequences of allowing mutagens to interact with it.

It has been interestingly different from other branches of toxicology in its development, for the concern about hazard started with the geneticists' theoretical knowledge of DNA and its functions, rather than with any observation of toxicological effect in man, although chemical carcinogenesis, of course, has a long history. Where these genetic effects have been sought they have been found, albeit not always in man. Moreover geneticists have developed the technology to enable DNA-damaging agents to be identified and studied in a routine practicable way, and this area constitutes the subject of this book.

Acknowledgement

I am grateful to Professor Paul Polani, FRS, for information on the nature and frequencies of genetic disease in man.

References

1. Yamasaki, E. and Ames, B. N. (1977). Concentration of mutagens from urine by adsorption with the non-polar resin XAD-2: Cigarette smokers have mutagenic urine. *Proc. Natl. Acad. Sci. USA*, **74**, 3555
2. Mau, G. and Netter, P. (1974). Die Auswirkungen des väterlichen Zigaretten-konsums auf die perinatale Sterblichkeit und die Missbildungshäufigkeit. *Dtsch Med. Wochenschr.*, **99**, 1113
3. Infante, P. F., Wagoner, J. K. and Waxweiler, R. J. (1976). Carcinogenic, mutagenic and teratogenic risks associated with vinyl chloride. *Mutat. Res.*, **41**, 131
4. Paddle, G. M. (1976). Genetic risks of vinyl chloride. *Lancet*, **May 15**, 1079
5. Infante, P. F., Wagoner, J. K., McMichael, A. J., Waxweiler, R. J. and Falk, H. (1976). Genetic risks of vinyl chloride. *Lancet*, **June 12**, 1289
6. Ad Hoc Committee (Cohen, E. N. *et al.*) (1974). Occupational disease among operating room personnel. *Anesthesiology*, **41**, 321
7. Ad hoc Committee (Cohen, E. N. *et al.*) (1975). A survey of anesthetic health hazards among dentists. *J. Am. Dent. Assoc.*, **90**, 1291
8. Bridges, B. A. (1976). Short-term screening tests for carcinogens. *Nature (London)*, **261**, 195
9. Doll, R. (1967). *Prevention of Cancer – Pointers for Epidemiology* (London: Whitefriars Press)
10. Benditt, E. P. (1977). The origin of atherosclerosis. *Sci. Am.*, **236**, 74
11. Evans, H. J. and O'Riordan, M. L. (1977). Human peripheral blood lymphocytes for the analysis of chromosome aberrations in mutagen tests. In: B. J. Kilbey, M. Legator, W. Nicholas and C. Ramel (eds.). *Handbook of Mutagenicity Test Procedures*, pp. 261–71 (Amsterdam: Elsevier/North Holland)
12. Strauss, G. H. and Albertini, R. J. (1977). 6-Thioguanine-resistant lymphocytes in human peripheral blood. In: D. Scott, B. A. Bridges and F. H. Sobels (eds.). *Progress in Genetic Toxicology*, pp. 327–34 (Amsterdam: Elsevier/North Holland)
13. Killian, D. J. and Picciano, D. (1976). Cytogenetic surveillance of industrial populations. In: A. Hollaender (ed.). *Chemical Mutagens: Principles and Methods for Their Detection, Vol. 4*, pp. 321–39 (New York: Plenum)
14. Lehmann, A. R. and Bridges, B. A. (1978). DNA repair. *Essays in Biochemistry*, **13**, 71
15. Arlett, C. F. and Lehmann, A. R. (1978). Human disorders showing increased sensitivity to the induction of genetic damage. *Ann. Rev. Genet.*, **12**, (In press)

2

The role of *Drosophila* in mutagen testing
C. Auerbach

Drosophila tests have an important, but somewhat special role in mutagen testing. First I must describe the essential features of the only test that really matters: the test for recessive sex-linked lethals. The terms describe the sex-linked mutations recorded as the result of the test, i.e. mutations on the X chromosomes, of which the female has two, while the male has only one. The second male sex chromosome is the Y, which carries very few genes. The mutations are lethal, that is, they kill the individual before it develops into a fly. Finally, they are recessive, in other words, they do not manifest themselves in the presence of the normal gene on the partner chromosome. Thus, a sex-linked recessive kills each male that carries it on his one X chromosome, but does not kill a female that carries it on only one of her two X chromosomes.

Figure 2.1 shows diagrammatically how the test is carried out. In the parental generation, the P_1 males are treated, the type of treatment depending on the type of risk to which humans may be exposed. Food additives and drugs will be added to the drinking water or the food of the flies or larvae; volatile substances will be administered as vapour or aerosol. No genetic effects can be expected to show up in the treated males themselves; these serve only as carriers of affected germ cells. They produce two types of spermatozoa: those containing the Y, and those containing

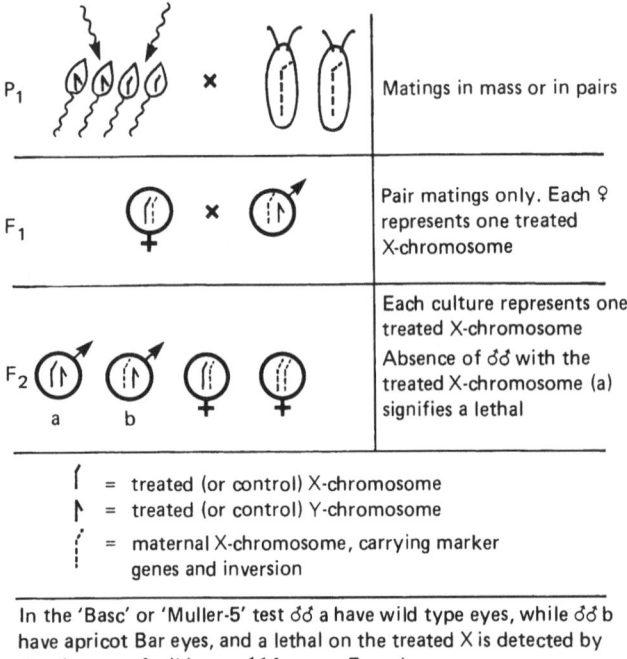

P_1	Matings in mass or in pairs
F_1	Pair matings only. Each ♀ represents one treated X-chromosome
F_2 a b	Each culture represents one treated X-chromosome Absence of ♂♂ with the treated X-chromosome (a) signifies a lethal

ʃ = treated (or control) X-chromosome
ʌ = treated (or control) Y-chromosome
ʄ = maternal X-chromosome, carrying marker genes and inversion

In the 'Basc' or 'Muller-5' test ♂♂ a have wild type eyes, while ♂♂ b have apricot Bar eyes, and a lethal on the treated X is detected by the absence of wild-type ♂♂ from an F_2 culture.

Figure 2.1   Test for sex-linked lethals in *Drosophila*

the X; only the latter are of interest for the test. The males are mated to untreated females all of whose eggs carry an untreated X. Suitable sex-linked genes, for example for body colour or eye colour, are used to distinguish between males with the treated and untreated X chromosomes. The first filial generation, the F_1, consists of males with the treated Y and females with the treated X. Because of the presence in them of the untreated X the females are viable whether or not they carry a sex-linked lethal. They are mated individually with any kind of suitable male, usually a brother. Each female represents one treated X chromosome; If this chromosome carries a lethal, all sons that inherit it will die and the female will have no sons with the treated X. Scoring the F_2 cultures consists of holding each vial against the light and looking for males with the treated X. Many young people can do this with the naked eye; others have to use a low-power binocular.

    The test is extremely simple and requires no previous training in biology, let alone genetics. Any normally intelligent and observant person can learn it in a few weeks. It is also practically free of personal error, for the absence of a whole class of flies from a culture can hardly be missed by anybody. The equipment, too, is very simple: a low-power binocular, an etherizing device for anaesthetizing flies, a brush for moving them about on a small china or glass tray, milk bottles for mass cultures, vials for individual cultures, metal trays for keeping the experimental vials in batches of, for example, 200, and a room kept at a moderately constant temperature around 25 °C with shelves for stacking the trays.

Now we come to those special features of the test that determine its usefulness in mutagen screening.

1. *Drosophila* is a eukaryotic animal, with typically eukaryotic chromosomes.

2. The test is applied to germ cells, not – as in many other systems – to somatic cells. Moreover, by mating treated males to a succession of females every few days, one can sample germ cells that, at the time of treatment, were in different stages of spermatogenesis. The first brood will be drawn from germ cells that were treated as spermatozoa; the last ones will be drawn from germ cells that were treated as spermatogonia. In man, spermatogonia – because of their long lifespan – are considered the cell type most at risk. It is therefore fortunate that in the *Drosophila* test we can examine specifically the response of spermatogonia to potential mutagens.

3. All sex-linked lethals are nuclear mutations; this follows from the fact that they occur on a specific chromosome and, at meiosis, segregate with this chromosome. In tests on micro-organisms and cell cultures, it is often difficult or even impossible to distinguish between true nuclear mutations, cytoplasmic mutations, and purely phenotypic changes.

The X chromosome forms one-fifth of the whole genome and, at a very conservative estimate, carries 500–600 genes capable of yielding lethal mutations. This has to be compared with the fact that in tests on micro-organisms or cell cultures one usually looks for mutations at only one or two loci. It is true that, quantitatively, this superiority of the *Drosophila* test is offset by the very much larger scale on which tests on micro-organisms and cell cultures can be carried out. Qualitatively, however, there remains the great advantage that differences between the responses of individual loci, well known from experiments with micro-organisms, will be swamped when several hundred loci are screened.

4. The greatest value lies in the fact that sex-linked lethals cover a whole range of different types of genetic damage. They may be internal changes in genes; they may also be deletions of a whole gene or of strings of

contiguous genes. It is the latter damage that, in my opinion, represents the greatest risk of mutagenic exposures for, while disturbed action or even complete lack of action of an individual gene may often not be particularly harmful, a string of several genes is almost certain to contain at least one whose action is required for survival. There are not many other systems in which tests for deletions can be carried out, and they are usually more complicated than a sex-linked lethal test. Moreover, deletions that can be scored in bacteria very probably have a different origin from those produced in eukaryotic chromosomes, which arise through loss of a small chromosome segment between two closely neighbouring breaks.

5. Finally, a very useful feature of the *Drosophila* tests became apparent in the course of mutagen screening. It is the possession, by *Drosophila*, of most of the enzymes that, in mammals, activate potential mutagens. Thus, activation by liver microsomes is not necessary, while phenobarbital seems to stimulate activation in *Drosophila* as it does in mammals.

I now come to the question of controls. It is here that *Drosophila*, in my opinion, occupies a very special position. It is considered mandatory that every mutation test should be accompanied by a so-called negative control, that is, by a mutation test on an untreated sample from the same population. This certainly applies to tests on micro-organisms and cell cultures, which will not only yield a certain number of new 'spontaneous' mutations in the controls, but also an unknown number, often quite large, of pre-existing mutations that have accumulated during previous growth of the culture. In *Drosophila* we need not worry about pre-existing lethals because the treated males are live males and therefore cannot carry a lethal. The only spontaneous mutations about which we have to worry are those arising *de novo* in the testes of these males. This is the so-called spontaneous mutation frequency of *Drosophila* males. The data on spontaneous mutation frequencies in wild-type laboratory stocks of *Drosophila* are voluminous; they have accumulated over many decades in many laboratories and, taken together, form a baseline which runs between 0.1% and 0.3%, with rare deviations to 0.5% or more, but hardly ever reaches 1% and never exceeds it. Moreover, in any particular laboratory, using its special strain of *Drosophila*, spontaneous mutation frequency remains remarkably constant over many years. In our laboratory it has always varied around 0.3%; in others it varies around 0.1%. With such a baseline at our disposal, it seems a waste of resources to carry out negative controls more than, say, once a year, and then only to establish whether the strain used has retained its customary mutation frequency. If, by some unlikely chance such as a mutator mutation, the strain should have become more mutable, one would have to replace it by another strain with normal spontaneous mutation frequency. There is one type of negative control which may sometimes be required. If treatment is carried out under conditions which by themselves may be suspected as mutagenic, such as the use of an untested carrier substance for an aerosol, mutations may have to be scored in flies that have been exposed to the experimental conditions in the absence of the substance under test. Whether one wants to use a positive control, that is, test the response of the strain to a known mutagen, is a matter of personal judgement. I personally feel sure that every *Drosophila* strain will respond to a good alkylating mutagen but, if one wants to test this, it can be done on quite a small scale.

The statistical treatment of the data will have to take account of the existing baseline of spontaneous mutation frequency. I think one should use quite rough estimates for deciding whether a result is positive, negative or doubtful; I would suggest calling any result of 1 % or more positive, any result of less than 0.5% negative, and any result in between, doubtful. Much more important than statistical significance of an individual test is consistency between replicates. In *Drosophila*, as in every other mutation test, replicates are indispensable. It is no good working with such large numbers that even a mutation frequency of 0.6% differs significantly from controls, unless the result can be repeated at least once, and this might require unmanageably large numbers. It is much better to make individual tests on moderately large numbers (say 2000 chromosomes per test) and to repeat them at least once, either with the same or with a different dose. A substance that, in two replicate tests, yields more than 1 % lethals can be confidently considered mutagenic for *Drosophila*. To me, this would make such a substance highly suspect for man and, unless there are very cogent reasons for using it in the human environment, I would condemn it on this basis alone without any further tests for mutation, although tests for chromosome breakage may still be desirable.

On the other hand, I do not feel that we can exonerate a substance that has given negative results in replicate *Drosophila* tests. Before giving such a substance clearance, corroborative evidence from other systems is required. Whether doubtful results should be repeated until the consistency of the data indicates a true mutagenic effect, depends on the time and money one wants to spend on *Drosophila* tests. There is, however, one possibility that can – and I think should – be examined in such cases: the possibility that the substance in question may produce only or mainly one-strand or otherwise delayed mutations. Even a strong mutagenic action of such a substance will be missed in the routine scoring of the F_2, but in the F_3 one-strand mutations and delayed mutations can be detected as easily as two-strand mutations are detected in F_2. From experiments of Dr Shukla in our laboratory it appears that hydroxylamine is such a substance: in all experiments in which lethals were scored in F_2, it gave at best doubtful results, but in two tests on F_3 the result was a clear positive. Since a lethal is equally deleterious, whether it has occurred as a one-strand or two-strand change, I feel that, for all substances that give negative or doubtful results in F_2, testing should be extended to F_3.

Figure 2.2 presents a tentative work schedule for one technician. I am sure it will need to be modified on the basis of experience, but I think that in its rough outline it is practicable. It takes account of three requirements:

Weeks	Chemicals									
	A		B		C		D		E	
	m	sc	m	sc	m	sc	m	sc	m	sc
1 + 2	m P_1	sc	m	sc	m	sc	m	sc	m	sc
3 + 4	F_1									
5 + 6	(F_2)	F_2 P_1								
7 + 8	(F_3)	F_1								
9 + 10	P_1		(F_2)	F_2 P_1						
11 + 12	F_1		(F_3)	F_1						
13 + 14	(F_2)	F_2 P_1		(F_2)	F_2 P_1			Recurrent	
15 + 16	(F_3) A	F_1		(F_3)	F_1			pattern	
17 + 18			(F_2)	F_2 P_1		(F_2)	F_2 P_1		
19 + 20			(F_3) B	F_1		(F_3)	F_1		

Figure 2.2 Suggested time schedule for routine testing of chemicals on *Drosophila* (see text for explanation)

testing of different germ cell stages as far back as spermatogonia (re-matings extending over about 10 days); one replication for each test, the two being done in sequence so that the results of the first can be taken into consideration when deciding on the dose used in the second; extension of the test to F_3 when the results in F_2 were negative or doubtful. I have divided the time into periods of two weeks, which is rather more than demanded by the first requirement. Each substance occupies two columns, one for the matings (m), the other for scoring (sc). The matings of F_2 and the scoring of F_3 have been put in brackets because they may not be necessary if the F_2 was positive. Once the recurrent pattern is established, one new substance is added every month, and one tested one is withdrawn. This makes it appear as if one technician could deal with twelve substances per year; but this is unrealistic. Not only are hitches sure to occur occa-sionally but more important is the fact that the technician will have holidays and will probably sometimes be on sick-leave. With a tight schedule like the one shown here, delay of the work will be considerably in excess of the actual period during which the technician is absent. I think it probable that one technician can deal with eight or nine substances per year. Employing a second technician will more than double this output because each of them can at least partially do the other's work during his absence. In fact, I think that two technicians plus one laboratory technician for medium-making and glassware-washing would be an ideal team for routine *Drosophila* tests, capable of dealing with about twenty sub-stances a year. In case of difficulties a trained geneticist should be available, although not necessarily in the same establishment.

Finally, I want to deal with the question of what position *Drosophila* should occupy in the tier system. In my opinion, this depends on our *a priori* expectations. As I see it, negative or doubtful results with *Drosophila* are not decisive evidence by themselves and require corroborative data from other systems. Therefore, if we have no reason to expect that a substance will be mutagenic, I should tend to leave the *Drosophila* test to a later tier or omit it altogether. On the contrary, a positive result in the *Drosophila* test – whether obtained in F_2 or F_3 – is extremely damning evidence. Therefore, if we have reasons to suspect that a substance will be mutagenic, I should use the *Drosophila* test very early in the tier; a positive result would make other tests for mutations unnecessary.

Let me give you a few examples for the efficacy of *Drosophila* tests in cases where mutagenicity of a substance was suspected on pharmacological, chemical or toxicological grounds. Mustard gas, the first strong chemical mutagen detected, was tested because of the pharmacological similarities between its effects and those of X-rays; the very first test yielded a staggeringly high frequency of sex-linked lethals. The related nitrogen mustard, which is equally effective in *Drosophila*, is only a weak mutagen for bacteria. We now know that mustard gas owes its mutagenic effect to alkylation of DNA. When other alkylating agents were tested on *Drosophila*, many were found to be strong mutagens. Heliotrine, an alkaloid found in ragwort, was tested on *Drosophila* because it produces liver damage in sheep; already the first experiments showed it to be a powerful mutagen. In bacteria it is at best very weakly mutagenic. Since a large number of substances will have to be tested yearly, it should not be difficult to find among them twenty which are suitable for early tests on *Drosophila*.

Discussion

Chairman: Professor B. N. Ames

Professor C. AUERBACH (Edinburgh): Was there not recently a report on negative results with captan *in vivo*?

Professor BRIDGES: There was a negative report for the dominant lethal test *in vivo* recently. The carcinogenicity test is an NCI test and has yet to be published – although I have seen it.

The reason for the negative dominant lethal test is very easily understandable in what is known about properties of captan. It is rather insoluble. When it dissolves it is quite unstable and it hydrolyses quite rapidly. The chances of its ever getting out of the gut where it is ingested are pretty remote, and it does not surprise me in the least that the only place that tumours can be found is the gut, which is where they were found in the mouse. I would think that the dominant lethal test, which is not a very sensitive test, is right on the borderline if it is to pick up anything.

Professor AUERBACH: So inhalation would be the real danger?

Professor BRIDGES: I have always maintained that inhalation of captan is the only mode of administration to man that is really worrying. It is sold as a very fine powder, with a lot of particles in the respirable range of less than 5–7 μm. It is an alkylating agent. It is known to be an alkylating agent, and it goes straight down into the lung where, unlike the gut, there is no vast concentration of thiol groups floating around in the lumen to mop up the active product.

I do think that if there is a hazard from captan, inhalation is the most likely cause.

QUESTION FROM THE FLOOR:
One way the industrial hygienist comes to suspect that there is a new carcinogen around is when some rather odd and unusual disease starts to turn up in his workforce. One wonders whether the same would hold true of the mutagenic effects of mutagens as opposed to their possible carcinogenic effects, and if there are indeed cases of an heritable clearly mutation-derived disease arising because of the action of a mutagen?

Professor BRIDGES: One would much sooner expect that than cancer. With cancer there is the whole overlying complexity of organ specificity. The metabolism of carcinogens is different in different organs of the body. This means that sometimes the carcinogen can be really quite specific in the organs that it attacks, like ethylamines in the bladder, or the vinyl chloride monomer in the liver. Where there is this specificity, a carcinogen can be detected. Where a carcinogen does not have such specificity, it will probably go undetected for ever, and we have to realize that – that there are probably a lot of them around that because they are not specific, they just raise the level of cancer in the population, but nothing abnormal is ever noticed.

If a bladder cancer comes along, or an angiosarcoma of the liver, an alert clinician, recognizing it as a rare cancer, might wonder about further cases in his practice, in the factory, in the neighbourhood. If he finds them he may have the first clue to an exposure. With genetic disease there is no organ specificity, but only the ovary and the testis, so there is no scope for different organs to metabolize the mutagen differently. The only way in which there might be specificity of genetic effects is if different genes responded differently. We do know enough to know that there is some gene specificity, but my reading of it is that it probably is not sufficient – ever – to enable one to expect a noticeable number of any particular type of abnormality.

Each individual abnormality, if it is a congenital abnormality, or a sex-linked disease, is rare enough anyway. The chance of picking up a second would require both that another one that was exposed was picked up *and* that they had the same change. I would have said that that is so unlikely that it would probably not be noticeable.

The answer in short is much less likelihood of a specific disease genetically related to a specific mutagen than there is with cancer and the carcinogen.

Professor D. V. PARKE (Guildford): When we talk about DNA, we normally think only of the nucleus. But there is DNA in the mitochondria, DNA in the endoplasmic reticulum.

The function of these is not fully known and I wonder if there is any information on damage to these other DNA's by chemical mutagens?

Professor BRIDGES: I am not aware of published work on the mito-chondrial DNA, for example, of mammals. If there is any, I have for-gotten about it. But mitochondrial DNA yeasts is certainly the subject of study – as a model system. There is now an accumulation of information about how mitochondrial DNA is repaired and mutated. It is only a matter of time before we can do similar things with mammalian cells – and answer the Professor's question.

QUESTION FROM THE FLOOR:
Professor Bridges mentioned cigarettes. Is anything known about the influence of additives in cigarettes. There are many additives in cigarettes and I wonder what is known of their influence?

Professor BRIDGES: I am sure there is a lot known. There is a lot of work being done using the *Salmonella* test investigating the mutagens that are present in cigarette smoke. There are a lot of mutagens. Some of them are very potent. There are also a number of synergistic agents which although not mutagenic in themselves are able to enhance the effect of the mutagens. The presence of mutagenic additives is known as well.

This work is taking place in Japan as well as in Professor Ames's own laboratories, and Professor Ames is perhaps better qualified to answer the question.

Professor B. N. AMES (Berkeley): Whenever anything is burnt, it produces some horrible mixture of chemicals, so almost any burnt substance, whether a car exhaust, a charcoal-broiled steak or cigarette smoke condensate is just chock full of all kinds of mutagens. I do not know whether the additives are doing something besides that, but there are plenty of mutagens as it is.

People may be slightly neglecting the effect of germ cell live mutations because people are very worried about cancer. One tends always to think about carcinogenesis, but it may be that germ cell line mutations are a more important public health problem than cancer, or at least equal to it. In micro-organisms, if a gene is mutated, one will see perhaps ten slightly damaged proteins that do not work very well for every mutation that completely destroys activity. Many of the effects of genes in people such as intelligence or fitness are the expression of many many genes, and it may be that the mutations seen in people are just a small percentage of the general effect, and that as the human mutation rate is increased, there may be all kinds of effects on general intelligence, or fitness, that are not perceived.

QUESTION FROM THE FLOOR:
One of the inevitable consequences of life is death, and death is frequently, although not invariably, preceeded by the ageing process – senescence. It is my understanding that when the ageing process is studied at the cellular level many changes are seen in chromosomes, genes and DNA that are similar to those that may be induced by environmental agents.

Would Professor Bridges enlarge on what he has said on the process of senescence, and whether there is any suggestion that senescence is environmentally induced rather than a simple consequence – as most of us have believed – of the process of time. As we grow older, our hair greys, our skin wrinkles, our teeth fall out, and whatever.

Professor BRIDGES: If a population is treated with chronic doses of a mutagen such as ionizing radiation then the lifespan is shortened. This is seen in animal studies. So one would expect that if DNA is damaged a little at a time, but for long enough, the organism will peg out rather sooner than it would do otherwise. But as to actual evidence for the involvement of environmental mutagens, or DNA-damaging agents as affecting senescence in man, there is no evidence that I would think work considering. It is a real working hypothesis. There are some people who believe that senescence is due to progressive damage to the DNA repair mechanisms, which in turn cause the DNA to fail to be repaired, and so some catastrophic situation is reached where the DNA cannot cope with the cell and the cell dies. But these are very controversial areas, and we ought to think of them as working hypotheses, fascinating ones.

Certainly the cellular models for ageing used in some laboratories – there are a number of us who are far from convinced that they are real models of ageing. They may be totally a laboratory artefact.

The whole area of ageing is fascinating, but still at that lovely realm of speculation where theories may be built up and tested if the right material can be found.

Professor AMES: One comment. On average the two-pack a day cigarette smoker lives 10 years less than the non-smoker. Some of that is due to lung cancer, but a lot is due to heart disease and other factors. It is a little hard to pin down all the specifics. It is very hard to get a grip on the ageing problem.

Professor BRIDGES: The crux I suppose is that with the smokers if the cancer is taken away, and the bronchitis, and the heart disease, is there anything left which is not specific but which causes them to die sooner. The answer to that is that there is no really clear evidence yet that there is. Of course epidemiological statistics have to be used, and that is not a good material for doing this sort of analysis.

QUESTION FROM THE FLOOR:
Professor Auerbach mentioned sex-linked lethals. Is there any virtue in using other *Drosophila* tests that she would recommend?

Professor C. AUERBACH (Edinburgh): No. If there is a positive result with the sex-linked lethals, then it is easy to test for chromosome breakage by doing a translocation test. It is not difficult. But I would then suggest testing for translocations in mammalian cells. There is no virtue in using *Drosophila* other than for the sex-linked lethal tests. Cytological tests are much better done on material which is closer to man, or even on mammalian cells. Usually dominant lethal tests are recommended. These are tests for hatchability. But they will be done anyway. With a new substance one must test for its toxicity and its toxicity will include effects on fertility. But the dominant lethal tests do not mean very much. There are so many reasons why the eggs may not hatch. I would only use the sex-linked lethal test because I think it has very great advantages.

QUESTION FROM THE FLOOR:
What would be the approximate cost to a company to have these tests?

Professor AUERBACH: I am not *au fait* with the figures. We have put together a project with Inveresk. We do not know whether it will be carried out. But the costing was not done by me. I am very bad at it. I think it is quite expensive.

The materials are very cheap. There is no need for a high-power microscope. Only a very low-power microscope is needed. The glassware is recycled. The only expensive material is the agar because there is 1 % or 2 % agar in the food. Otherwise the materials are not expensive. In the original outlay the expense will be to have a room in which the cultures can be kept at a fairly constant temperature. It does not need to be very constant, but between 20 and 23 °C. Otherwise there will be such a delay in development. That would be the initial outlay. After that the outlay is very small, but there is then the question of the technicians, and of expensive scientists with the skill to interpret the results.

SECTION TWO

Bacterial Tests for Mutagenesis

3

A strategy to minimize human exposure to environmental chemicals causing cancer and genetic birth defects*

B. N. Ames

DAMAGE TO DNA BY ENVIRONMENTAL MUTAGENS CAUSES CANCER AND GENETIC BIRTH DEFECTS

Damage to DNA (the genetic material in our cells) appears to be the most likely cause of most cancer and genetic birth defects, and may contribute to heart disease and ageing as well. These are the major diseases now confronting our society: currently almost one-fourth of us will develop cancer, while 5–10% of our children are born with birth defects.

Environmental mutagens, both natural and man made, appear to be the agents causing much of this genetic damage. Damage to the DNA of our germ cells, those cells forming the sperm and eggs, results in genetic defects that show up in our children and in future generations. Somatic mutation, or damage to the DNA of the other cells of the body, can give rise to cancerous cells by changing the normal cellular mechanisms, coded

*This paper has been adapted from a California Policy Seminar Series Monograph, Institute of Governmental Studies, University of California, Berkeley 94720 (1978).

for in the DNA, that control and prevent cell multiplication. Many mutagens are present among the natural chemicals in our diet; among man-made chemicals to which we are exposed, such as industrial chemicals, pesticides, hair dyes, cosmetics, and drugs; and in complex mixtures such as cigarette smoke and contaminants in the air we breathe and the water we drink.

A variety of evidence supports the hypothesis that most cancer is caused by environmental factors[1,2]. Incidence rates for certain types of cancer in different parts of the world, particularly among immigrants, suggest most cancer is environmental, not genetic. For example, in Japan there is an extremely low rate of breast and colon cancer and a high rate of stomach cancer, whereas in the United States the reverse is true. When Japanese migrate to the United States, within a generation or two they show the high colon and breast cancer rates and low stomach cancer rates characteristic of other Americans.

In addition, the list of chemicals (and radiation) that have been impli-cated in causing human cancer is steadily lengthening despite the diffi-culties in human epidemiology. Among these mutagens/carcinogens are cigarette smoke tar, vinyl chloride, *bis*-chloromethyl ether, coal tar, aflatoxin (a mould product), β-naphthylamine and benzidine (aniline dye precursors), ultraviolet light, and X-rays. Even the physical carcinogen asbestos has recently been shown to be a mutagen; asbestos needles appear to pierce animal cells and cause chromosomal abnormalities[2].

IDENTIFYING MUTAGENS AND CARCINOGENS

Identifying the mutagens and carcinogens causing cancer in people is tremendously difficult owing to a long lag period of 20–30 years for the appearance of most types of human cancer following exposure to a carcinogen. This is dramatically illustrated in the case of cigarette smoking (Figure 3.1). Men started smoking cigarettes about 1900, but the resulting increase in lung cancer did not appear until 20–25 years later. Similary women started smoking in appreciable numbers about the time of the Second World War, and now the lung cancer rate for women is climbing rapidly. This same 20-year lag has been shown to apply for most types of cancer caused by the atomic bomb and for cancer in factory workers exposed to a variety of chemicals. Cigarette smoking has been much easier to identify as a cause of cancer than the usual environmental carcinogen because there is a clear control group of non-smokers and it causes a characteristic type of cancer (of the lung) that is infrequent in the control

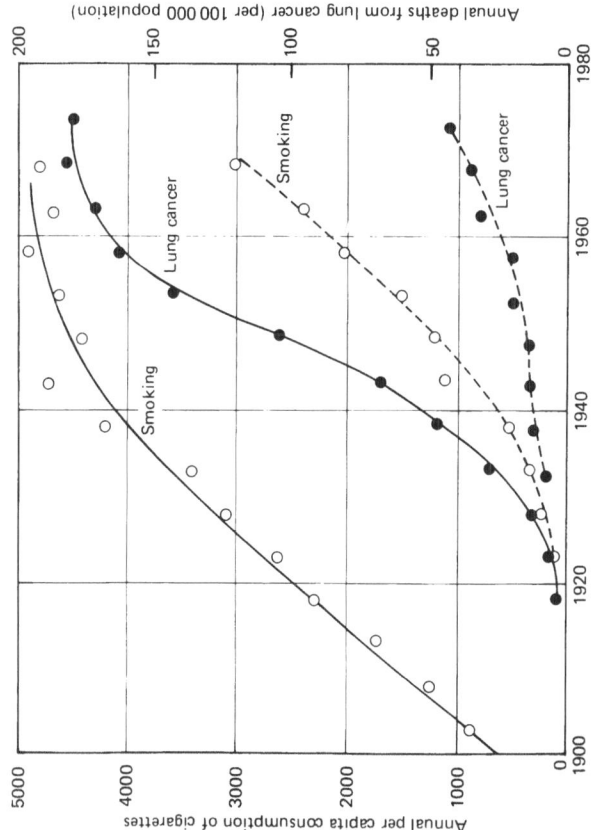

Figure 3.1 Cigarette smoking and lung cancer are unmistakably related, but the nature of the relation remained obscure because of the long latent period between the increase in cigarette consumption and the increase in the incidence of lung cancer. The data are for England and Wales. In men (solid line) smoking began to increase at the beginning of the twentieth century, but the corresponding trend in deaths from lung cancer did not begin until after 1920. In women (dotted line) smoking began later, and lung cancers are only now appearing (from J. Cairns (1975), *The Cancer Problem*, copyright Scientific American, Inc. All rights reserved)

group. However, with most environmental chemicals, such as the Japanese food additive AF-2 (discussed later) or vinyl chloride in spray cans, there is no clearcut unexposed group; should certain carcinogens cause small increases in breast cancer or other common types of cancer, it will be even more difficult to show cause and effect, though the number of individuals affected might be large.

Human genetic defects are not easy to monitor or to attribute to a specific cause by epidemiology; thus a considerable increase in birth defects (exceeding the current rate of 5–10% among births) could easily go unnoticed. Moreover, many consequences of a general increase in gene mutations in the germ line are subtle, such as decreased intelligence or fitness. For example, a chemical mutagen and carcinogen – the agricultural pesticide dibromochloropropane (DBCP) – was recently taken off the market after it was discovered, somewhat by accident, that many DBCP workers had become sterile after exposure to it. DBCP might also cause a variety of genetic abnormalities among the offspring of workers who were able to conceive. If the sterility had not been connected with the occupational exposure, thus alerting us to the dangers of DBCP, it seems doubtful that genetic abnormalities and cancer that might occur years later would be connected to the earlier exposure.

NEW CHEMICALS IN OUR ENVIRONMENT

Clearly, many more chemicals will be added to the current list of human mutagens and carcinogens. It has been estimated that over 50 000 chemicals with significant production are currently used in commerce and close to 1000 new ones are introduced each year[3,4]. Only a small fraction of these chemicals – from flame retardants in our children's pyjamas to pesticides accumulating in our body fat – were tested for carcinogenicity or mutagenicity before their use. In the past this problem has been largely ignored, and even very high production chemicals, with extensive human exposure, were produced for decades before adequate carcinogenicity or mutagenicity tests were done. Such chemicals include vinyl chloride (5 billion lb/yr, USA) and 1,2-dichloroethane (ethylene dichloride, 8 billion lb/yr, USA) (Figure 3.2), and a host of high-production pesticides that have only recently been shown to be carcinogenic and mutagenic.

Even if we could easily identify new hazardous chemicals by human epidemiology, people would already have been exposed for decades, and the discovery would be too late for those exposed. This happened with vinyl chloride: it was used in millions of spray cans and in foods packaged in

PVC (polyvinyl chloride) containers for years before cancer was observed in factory workers exposed to it. A 20- to 30-year lag time is observed for the appearance of cancer after exposure to chemicals such as cigarette smoke condensate (Figure 3.1). The tremendous increase in production of chemicals, such as vinyl chloride, that started in the mid-1950s (Figure 3.2) may result in a steep increase in human cancer if many of these thousands

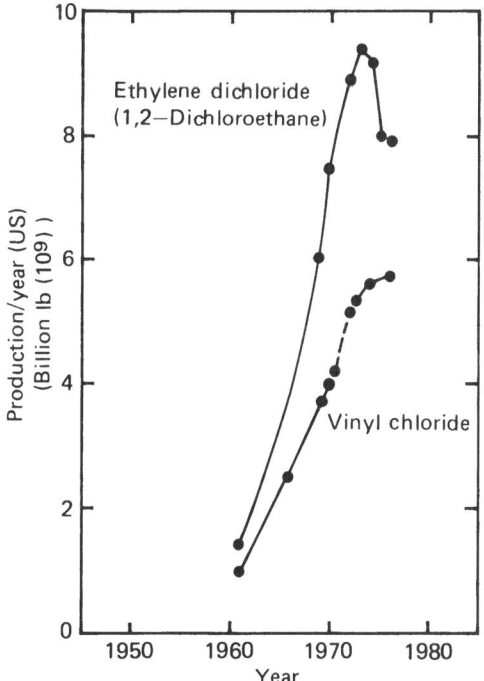

Figure 3.2   Production of two mutagens/carcinogens with widespread human exposure: ethylene dichloride and vinyl chloride (production data from 'Top-50 Chemicals' issues of *Chemical and Engineering News*). Approximately 100 billion lb of ethylene dichloride and over 50 billion lb of vinyl chloride have been produced since 1960. Ethylene dichloride is a volatile liquid that is the precursor of vinyl chloride and is also used extensively as a fumigant, solvent, petrol additive (200 million lb/yr), and metal degreaser. Ethylene dichloride was first shown to be a mutagen in *Drosophila* in 1960[5,6], and later in barley and *Salmonella*, but this fact has been ignored. The first adequate cancer test in animals has just been completed by the National Cancer Institute (September 1978) and is positive in both sexes of both rats and mice. Vinyl chloride gas is used to make polyvinyl chloride (PVC; vinyl) plastic. It was shown to be a carcinogen in rats and in people in the mid-1970s, and a mutagen in *Salmonella* and other systems shortly afterwards

of chemicals are indeed powerful mutagens and carcinogens with wide-spread human exposure.

HUMAN EXPOSURE TO MAN-MADE CHEMICALS

We are exposed intermittently to a wide variety of dietary mutagenic and carcinogenic chemicals, as well as to such man-made ones as chloroform in toothpaste, cough medicine, and water; vinyl chloride in spray cans; and aromatic amines in hair dyes. There are other carcinogens to which we are continuously exposed: those that have accumulated in our body fat, such as flame retardants, polychlorinated biphenyls (PCBs), and a wide variety of persistent, chlorinated pesticides. These substances are continuously present in our cell membranes, and the dose levels are disturbing. Table 3.1

Table 3.1   Chlorinated pesticides and PCBs in Canadian human fat (average of 168 samples. Almost all have been shown to be carcinogens).

Compound	μg/kg Wet weight mean	Per cent of samples containing residues
PCB	907	100
Hexachlorobenzene	62	100
BHC (Lindane)	65	88
Oxychlordane	55	97
Trans-Nonachlor	65	99
Heptachlor epoxide	43	100
Dieldrin	69	100
P.P′–DDE	2 095	100
O.P′–DDT	31	63
P.P′–TDE	6	26
P.P′–DDT	439	100

From J. Mes, D. S. Campbell, R. N. Robinson, and D. J. A. Davies, (1977). *Bull. Environ, Contam. Toxicol.*, **17**, 196

shows some chlorine-containing chemicals found in human body fat: almost all are known carcinogens. Tables 3.2 and 3.3 shows the levels of some of these same pesticides in human mothers' milk. The chemicals that were assayed for in these studies are only some of those that have accumulated in people. Carcinogens such as toxaphene, kepone, mirex, and other major pesticides are also accumulating in the food chain. In addition, a wide variety of industrial chemicals, as yet untested for carcinogenicity, are likely to be carcinogens, by analogy with similar carcinogenic chemicals, and to bioaccumulate in people. These include the notorious polybrominated biphenyls (PBBs), about 500 lb of which were accidentally mixed into Michigan cattle feed, causing an upheaval in the dairy farms in the state; millions of pounds of this man-made chemical are in the environment and may eventually haunt us as the polychlorinated biphenyls (PCBs) have[7]. Pentachlorophenol, the main wood preservative, is found in humans at appreciable levels[8]. Among the compounds in the expired air of normal adults are five different chlorinated compounds, including dichlorobenzene (used as moth crystals)[9].

Table 3.2   Some pesticides in human milk, 1400 U.S. women (1976 EPA data)*

Pesticide	Levels detected ($\mu g/kg$) on a fat basis Mean of positive	Maximum	% Positive
DDE	3 521	214 167	100
DDT	529	34 369	99
Dieldrin	164	12 300	81
Heptachlor epoxide	91	2 050	64
Oxychlordane	96	5 700	63
BHC (Lindane)	183	9 217	87
PCBs	2 076	12 600	30*

* From S. G. Harris and J. H. Highland (1977), *Birthright Denied* (Washington, D.C.: Environmental Defense Fund). (PCBs 1038 women, EPA 1977, >1100 $\mu g/kg$ fat; 99% of women had detectable PCBs

Table 3.3   Average daily intake of pesticides by a nursing infant (1976 EPA data)*

Pesticide	WHO acceptable intake ($\mu g/kg/day$)	Actual intake ($\mu g/kg/day$) Average	Maximum
DDE	5	13.8	38
Dieldrin	0.1	0.92	73
Heptachlor epoxide	0.5	0.52	12

* From S. G. Harris and J. H. Highland (1977), *Birthright Denied* (Washington, D.C.: Environmental Defense Fund)

Organic chemicals containing chlorine and bromine are not used in natural mammalian biochemical processes and were not normally present in the human diet until the onset of the modern chemical age. An extremely high percentage of chlorinated and brominated chemicals are carcinogens in animal cancer tests and mutagens in short-term tests. In contrast, among those chemicals without chlorine and bromine, a low percentage has been found to be mutagenic or carcinogenic.

IS THERE A SAFE DOSE OF MUTAGENS AND CARCINOGENS?

Some say there is a safe dose for each carcinogen and that we should not be concerned about the exposure of a large population to a low dose. Though we have no firm answer, several arguments suggest that this is not likely to be the general case.

1. The best dose–response information is the human data on cancer incidence *v.* cigarette smoking (Figure 3.3), which does not support the hypothesis of a threshold or safe level. Studies on humans exposed to

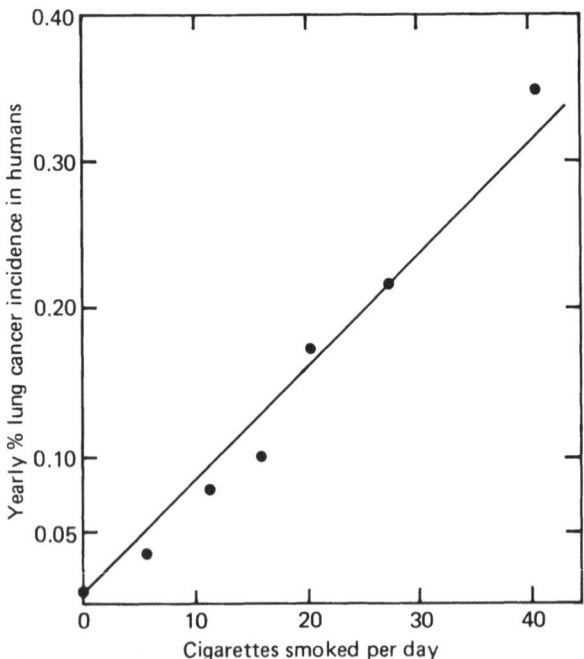

Figure 3.3 Dose–response curve on cancer incidence *v.* cigarettes smoked. (From R. Doll, in *Oncology 1970;* R. L. Clark *et al.* eds. Year Book Medical Publishers Inc. Chicago, Ill. 1971 pp. 1–28)

radiation also provide no support for a safe dose. It is impossible to get statistically significant information at low dose levels from animal cancer experiments, in which only a few hundred animals are exposed to the chemical.

2. Most carcinogens appear to have the same mechanism of action as mutagens, and thus it appears likely that the doses of the many carcinogens to which we are exposed will have an additive effect. We are high up on the human dose–response curve (currently about 25% of us will get cancer), and it seems reasonable that these increments of environmental carcinogens will increase risk linearly[10,11]. It seems prudent to assume, until shown otherwise experimentally, that there is no safe dose of a carcinogen. There are still risk-benefit considerations, however, and few human activities are without some risk. Individuals may be willing to accept low, and even high, risks: a two-packet-a-day smoker (40 cigarettes) lives on the average about 8 years less than does a non-smoker.

ANIMAL CANCER TESTS

A key method for detecting carcinogens is the animal bioassay, usually with rats and mice. The dozen or so organic chemicals known to cause cancer in humans also cause cancer in experimental animals when adequately tested. Those chemicals to which we are exposed in appreciable amounts should be screened in animal tests. The National Cancer Institute is testing a number of the key industrial compounds to which many humans are being exposed. One limitation of animal cancer tests, however, is their sensitivity. An environmental carcinogen causing cancer in 1% of 100 million people would result in a million cases of cancer. To detect a chemical causing cancer in 1% of the test animals, we would have to use 10 000 rats or mice. This enormous animal experiment would be necessary to overcome inherent statistical limitations, where an increase in the number of tumours has some probability of being due to chance. Yet in fact, a group size of only 50 mice or rats of each sex at each of two doses is the usual size of the most thorough cancer experiments; larger groups are too expensive. Thus, in order to demonstrate the safety of a chemical for millions of people by using only a few hundred test animals (there is no way this can be done with complete satisfaction), the animals are exposed to as high a dose as possible without actually killing them. The high doses are used to try to overcome the statistical problems inherent in the small sample size.

Another limitation in testing for carcinogens using animals is the enormity of the undertaking. There are not enough pathologists to read the slides even if we decided to test the thousand or so new chemicals introduced in commerce each year, not to mention the problem of coping with a backlog of the approximately 50 000 commercial chemicals that lack adequate testing for cancer in animals.

A further limitation is that chemical and drug companies need to have a method for weeding out hazardous chemicals while they are still under development and while alternatives can be chosen. Currently, many chemicals undergo a long-term animal test, if they are tested at all, after millions of dollars have been invested in them. Animal cancer tests are too expensive (approximately $300 000 per chemical) and take too long (two to three years) for the testing of all the new chemicals under development. They can only be used for the chemicals with major human exposure.

Also needed is a less expensive and quicker test for identifying the carcinogens in the many complex mixtures of chemicals that surround us, such as cigarette smoke, impurities in water and air, natural carcinogens in our diet, and complex industrial products. Animal tests are usually not suitable as bioassays for identifying the active agent in a complex mixture because of the time and expense.

THE *SALMONELLA*/MAMMALIAN LIVER TEST

Over the past 14 years we have developed a simple test for identifying chemical mutagens and have shown that almost all organic chemical carcinogens are mutagens[12-15]. The method is being widely used to detect environmental carcinogens as mutagens. This test, and other short-term tests that have been developed, should enable society to solve some of the problems that could not be approached using human epidemiology or animal cancer tests.

This work started as an offshoot from our basic research on the molecular biology of *Salmonella* bacteria. We were studying how genes are switched on and off in bacteria in response to the presence of nutrients in the growth medium. During the course of this work, we were mutating bacteria so that they could no longer make the amino acid histidine, a nutrient required for bacterial growth. We also had a large collection of histidine-requiring bacterial mutants made by Professor P. E. Hartman of Johns Hopkins University. It occurred to us in 1964 that it would be interesting to set up a test system for detecting mutagens using these bacteria. The genetic material, DNA, is the same in all living things, including bacteria. One can easily study mutagens in bacteria because a billion bacteria can be added to a single petri plate, on which the descendants of a single bacterium form a visible colony in about one day.

Our test detects mutagens by means of their ability to damage DNA and we have shown that about 90% of organic carcinogens can be detected as mutagens. DNA damage is measured using special strains of *Salmonella* bacteria in combination with homogenized liver tissue from rats (tissue homogenates from human autopsy material or from other mammals can also be used). The compound to be tested, about one billion bacteria of a particular tester strain (several different histidine-requiring mutants are used), and homogenized liver are combined on a petri dish and after incubation as body temperature (37 °C) for 2 days, the number of bacterial colonies is recorded. Each colony (a *revertant* colony) is composed of the descendants of a bacterium that has been mutated from a defective histidine gene to a functional one. Because of the ideas and work of Boyland, Magee, the Millers, the Weisburgers, and other workers[2] the understanding has developed that many carcinogens must be converted by enzymes in liver or other tissues to an active form that is the true carcinogen (and mutagen). We thus added mammalian liver tissue to the test to provide a first approximation of mammalian metabolism.

Results with Mutagens

Figures 3.4 and 3.5 show examples of the type of results obtained. In the 'spot test' (Figure 3.5), a small amount of the chemical to be tested is placed in the centre of the dish, the chemical diffuses out into the agar, and revertant colonies appear in the diffusion zone. The spot test is somewhat limited in sensitivity, but it is extremely rapid.

Normally, one tests individual doses of a chemical in the more sensitive plate test, and quantitative dose–response curves are generated as shown in Figure 3.5. These curves are almost always linear, which suggests that there is no threshold, or safe dose, for a mutagen. Most mutagens are detected at very low doses, in some cases in nanogram amounts.

The simplicity, sensitivity, and accuracy of this test for screening large numbers of environmental sources of potential carcinogens has resulted in its current use in over 1000 government, industrial, and academic laboratories throughout the world. A number of companies have made important economic decisions on the basis of the test. DuPont has recently decided (at considerable economic loss) not to use two Freon propellants in spray cans (they were available replacements for the Freon that is damaging the ozone layer) because they were mutagens.

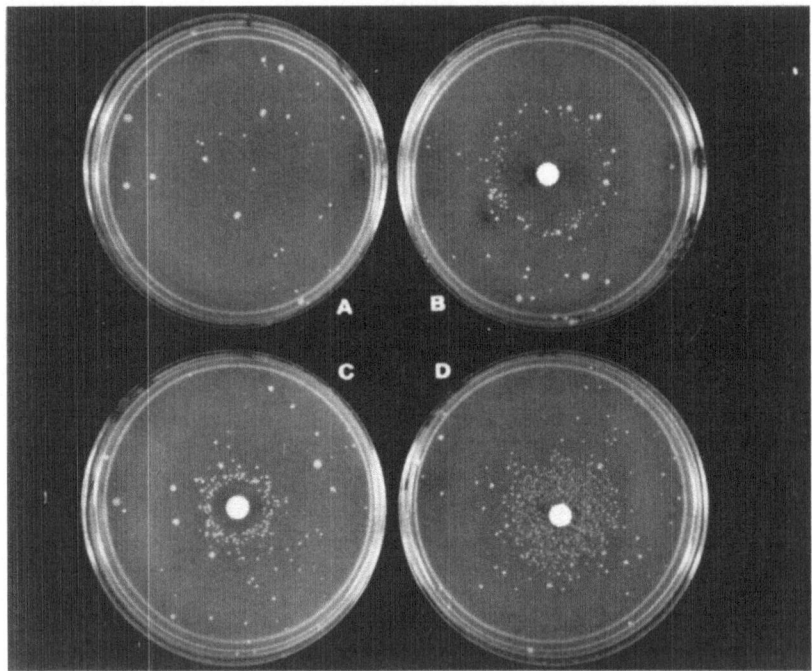

Figure 3.4 The 'spot test'. Each petri plate contains, in a thin overlay of top agar, the tester strain TA98 and, in the cases of plates C and D, a liver microsomal activation system (S-9 Mix). Mutagens were applied to 6 mm filter-paper discs, which were then placed in the centre of each plate: (A) spontaneous revertants; (B) the Japanese food additive furylfuramide (AF-2) (1 μg); (C) the mould carcinogen aflatoxin B_1 (1 μg); (D) 2-aminofluorene (10 μg). Mutagen-induced revertants appear as a ring of colonies around each disc. (Reprinted, with permission, from B. N. Ames, J. McCann, and E. Yamasaki (1975). *Mutation Res.*, **31**, 347)

Validation

We have validated the test for the detection of carcinogens as mutagens by examining over 300 chemicals reported as carcinogens or non-carcinogens in animal carcinogenicity experiments[13-15]. The results show that almost all (90%: 158/176) of these chemical carcinogens are mutagenic in the *Salmonella* test. The percentage of carcinogens detectable would, of course, depend on how representative any particular list of carcinogens was of those existing in the real world. For this reason we also examined

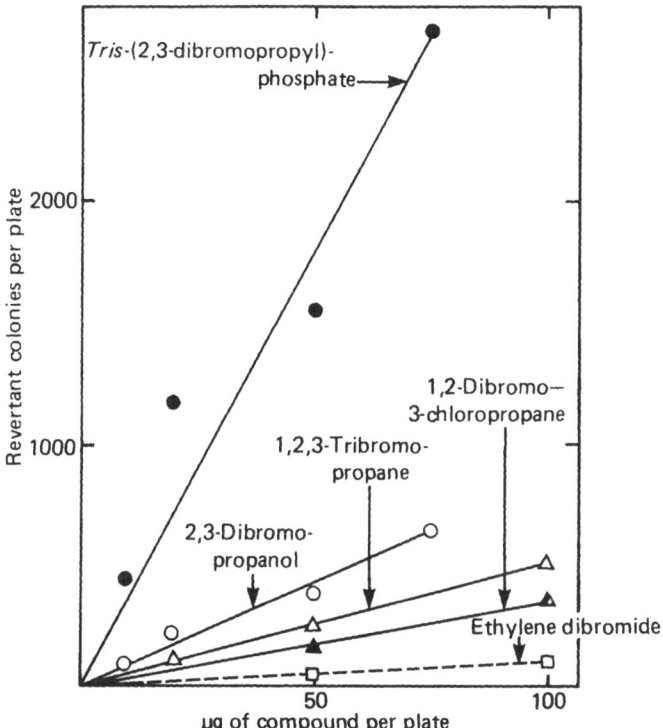

Figure 3.5 The flame retardant *tris*- (2,3-dibromopropyl) phosphate and the pesticide dibromochloropropane were in the presence of rat liver homogenate. All compounds were tested on *Salmonella* strain TA100. The amount of the industrial chemical ethylene dibromide added was ten times that indicated on the scale. (Reprinted, with permission, from A. Blum and B. N. Ames. (1977). *Science*, **195**, 17; copyright 1977 by the American Association for the Advancement of Science)

the organic chemicals known or suspected as human carcinogens and found that almost all (16/18) were mutagens in the test[15]. Nevertheless, it is important to emphasize that some important carcinogens[15] do not show up in the test, and that even with test improvements some carcinogens will never be detected because they are not acting through a direct interaction with DNA.

Thus, almost all carcinogens are mutagens, and the converse also appears to be true: mutagens are carcinogens with few (if any) adequately documented exceptions. We found that almost all (95/108) 'non-carcinogens' tested were not mutagenic and those few that were may in fact be carcinogens, but were not detected as such due to the statistical limitations of animal carcinogenicity tests[13-15].

Our test system has been independently validated, with similar results, in studies by Imperial Chemical Industries and by the National Cancer Institute in Tokyo.

Further validation is offered by several cases involving extensive human exposure, where chemicals initially detected as mutagens have subsequently been found to be carcinogens. One incident involved the food additive, AF-2 (furylfuramide)[16,17], which was used extensively in Japan from 1965 until recently as an antibacterial additive in a wide variety of common food products such as soybean curd and fish sausage. It showed no carcinogenic activity in tests on rats in 1962 and on mice in 1971. In 1973, however, Japanese scientists found it to be highly mutagenic in a strain of *Escherichia coli* bacteria (it was also found to be extraordinarily potent in reverting our *Salmonella* tester strain TA100 (see Figure 3.4)). The mutagenic activity of this chemical in food was such that one could easily demonstrate the mutagenicity of a slice of fish sausage put on a petri plate. It was subsequently examined in higher (eukaryotic) organisms and found to be mutagenic in yeast and *Neurospora*, to cause chromosome breaks in human white blood cells, and more recently to mutate embryos when even low doses were fed to pregnant Syrian hamsters[17]. Animal tests for carcinogenicity, more extensive than the previous ones, were initiated, and these tests have recently shown that AF-2 is, in fact, a carcinogen in rats and mice. As a consequence, the Japanese government prohibited the use of AF-2 as a food additive, and all products containing AF-2 were removed from the market. Since AF-2 had already been tested for carcinogenicity in two animal systems and found negative, it is unlikely that further tests would have been conducted if it had not been shown to be mutagenic. Any deleterious effects of AF-2 on the Japanese population would not have been evident for decades, and it is possible that a catastrophe may have been avoided by the early detection of this carcinogen with a simple bacterial mutagenicity test. Unfortunately, for the past eight years, the Japanese people have consumed relatively large amounts of AF-2; it is still too early to predict the consequences of this exposure.

Ethylene dichloride, a nine-billion-lb-a-year chemical, shown in Figure 3.2, has been shown previously to be a mutagen in the fruit fly, *Drosophila*, in barley, and in *Salmonella* and has now been found to be a carcinogen.

Another example of a carcinogen initially detected as a mutagen is 1,2-dibromoethane (ethylene dibromide), a widely used industrial chemical and gasoline additive, which was detected as a mutagen in several microbial systems (including the *Salmonella* test [see Figure 3.5]) over eight years ago[3]. It was tested for carcinogenicity and found positive in 1973. One hopes that the 400 million lb per year used in the United States are treated with the respect such a potent carcinogen deserves. It is closely related in structure to the pesticide dibromochloropropane (also a mutagen and a carcinogen), discussed previously.

Another related dibromo chemical, *tris*- (2,3-dibromopropyl) phosphate, commonly called 'Tris', the main flame-retardant in children's polyester pyjamas, is a potent mutagen in our test system, as are its metabolically produced breakdown product, dibromopropanol, and its impurity, the carcinogen dibromochloropropane (Figure 3.5)[18,19]. Fifty million children wore sleepwear that contained this material, at about 5% of the weight of the fabric. We argued that Tris would pose a serious hazard to children because non-polar (relatively fat–soluble and water–insoluble) chemicals such as these are generally absorbed through human skin at appreciable rates. Since its detection as a mutagen in *Salmonella*, it has been shown to be active in a number of short-term tests: it is a potent mutagen in *Drosophila*, it interacts with human DNA, and it damages mammalian chromosomes. The compound has recently been tested at the National Cancer Institute, and the results show that Tris is a potent carcinogen in both rats and mice. It has also been shown, like dibromochloropropane, to cause sterility in animals. It has now been banned for use in sleepwear. We have recently shown that a Tris metabolite, dibromopropanol, is present in the urine of children wearing Tris-treated sleepwear.

Studies in this laboratory have shown that most common hair dyes are mutagens[20]; 89% (150/169) of commercial oxidative-type (hydrogen peroxide) hair dye formulations were mutagenic, and of the 18 components of these hair dyes, eight were mutagenic. Most semi-permanent hair dyes tested were also shown to be mutagenic. Hair dye components are known to be absorbed through the skin, yet very few of the hair dyes or their components have ever been tested adequately for carcinogenicity. Since the work on mutagenicity in *Salmonella*, a number of these ingredients have been shown to be mutagens in other short-term tests for mutagenicity. Several of the chemicals are being tested at the National Cancer Institute and now appear to be carcinogens. About 25 million people (mostly women) dye their hair in the United States, and the hazard could be considerable if these chemicals are mutagenic and carcinogenic in humans.

The sensitivity of the *Salmonella*/mammalian liver assay makes it useful as a tool for rapidly obtaining information about the mutagenic and potential carcinogenic activity of complex mixtures, where it can be used as an assay to identify the mutagenic components of the mixtures. A detailed study, for example, has been made of the mutagenic activity of cigarette smoke condensate and 12 standard smoke condensate fractions[21]. (In the test, the condensate from less than 0.01 cigarette could easily be detected.)

We have recently developed a simple method for examining human urine in our test system and have found mutagens in the urine of cigarette smokers but not in the urine of non-smokers[22].

OTHER SHORT-TERM TESTS

Since our development of the *Salmonella* test and the demonstration that almost all carcinogens are mutagens, there has been a tremendous resurgence of interest in other short-term test systems for measuring mutagenicity. Many such systems have been developed and some, including the use of animal cells in tissue culture and cytogenetic damage in cells in tissue culture, are quite promising and have been validated with a reasonable number of chemicals. In addition, a number of the old systems, such as mutagenicity testing in *Drosophila*, have become much more sophisticated (the first mutagens known, such as X-rays and mustard gas, were first identified in *Drosophila* before they were known to be carcinogens). In addition, the development of several tissue-culture systems with animal cells, having as an end point the 'transformation' of the cells to a tumour cell, are an important advance.

No one of these short-term tests, however, is completely ideal; for example, most tests using animal cells in culture require the addition of liver homogenate, just as our bacterial test does, because the animal cells useful for these tests are not capable of metabolizing all foreign chemicals to active mutagenic forms. The short-term systems that are being validated (none have been validated as extensively as *Salmonella*) seem to be effective in detecting known carcinogens. Because each system detects a few carcinogens that others do not, the idea of a battery of short-term tests is now favoured.

In the case of a substance like Tris, or the food additive AF-2, the combination of a widespread human exposure to the chemical and a positive result in a number of short-term tests should have been sufficient evidence to stop its use, considering that alternatives were available. Yet Tris and AF-2 were not removed from the market until the results from animal cancer tests indicated that they were carcinogens. It is becoming apparent that a positive result in many of these short-term test systems is meaningful, and that the systems may not only be a complement to animal cancer testing but may also provide much additional toxicological information as well. Animal cancer tests have their own limitations.

A number of tests with rodents are being developed to examine mutagenic damage in cells in the whole animal. (A direct measure of mutagenic activity in animals can be made by studying the progeny for genetic birth defects, but this is even more cumbersome and expensive than an animal cancer test, and it is hardly ever performed.) There are simple methods for looking at sterility or defective sperm in animals and because of the discovery that dibromochloropropane caused sterility in workers, interest in these methods should increase.

CARCINOGENIC POTENCY AND HUMAN RISK ASSESSMENT

There is human exposure to a large number of environmental carcinogens, both manmade and natural. Many of these chemicals are quite useful, and it is clearly impractical to ban every carcinogen. We must have some way of setting priorities for regulation of these chemicals, and this requires an assessment of human risk, a difficult and complex problem.

We believe it is important for the assessment of human risk to have knowledge of carcinogenic potency, which can be accomplished in part through a quantitative analysis of animal cancer tests. We (Sawyer, Hooper, Friedman, and Ames) have been working on the potency problem for over a year (following the lead of M. Meselson[23] and collaborating with R. Peto on the theoretical aspects), and are nearing completion of the first stage of our analysis of 1000 published animal cancer tests in which the dose is given continuously for the lifetime of the animal by feeding.

Our results to date show that it is essential to consider carcinogens in more quantitative terms. We have shown that the potency of carcinogens (the TD_{50}, the daily dose required to produce cancer in half of the animals) can vary over a million-fold. Such a range of potency must be considered in assessing the hazard of chemicals for man. This quantitative analysis of carcinogenic potency for all the cancer tests in the scientific literature that are suitable for calculation is almost complete. The results should be useful for the determination of:

1. Which chemicals, among the thousands of carcinogens to which people are exposed, present the greatest human hazard and require the most immediate attention. This setting of priorities also requires an estimate of the amount of human exposure to a given chemical – information that is often available or can be obtained.

2. The allowable exposure levels for carcinogens for workers or the general population.

3. The significance of negative cancer tests. Each particular cancer test has a limit of sensitivity (because of dose level and other factors) and can detect only those carcinogens having potencies above a certain level. Because cancer tests vary enormously in sensitivity, rather than using the quantitatively meaningless term *non-carcinogen*, we must express the results of a negative cancer test by assigning the chemical a maximum potency value. For human risk assessment, it is essential to know the maximum potency values for non-carcinogens.

4. To what extent carcinogenic potency is, or is not, species and sex specific, and which animal species and strain is the best model for humans for each particular class of carcinogens. Our analysis so far indicates that potency values do not vary much for a given chemical when comparing males and females and that, with a few exceptions, values for rats and mice are quite similar.

5. The relation of carcinogenic potency to potency as measured in many short-term tests, such as the *Salmonella* mutagenicity test. It is clear that mutagenicity tests also show a tremendous range in potency – there is about a million-fold range in *Salmonella*.

We believe that these applications of the potency scale can be applied to current problems. One example can be used to illustrate the immediate value of the scale. The pesticide dibromochloropropane was used at a level of about ten million lb per year in the United States. In 1961 it was shown to cause sterility and testicular atrophy in animals[24]; in 1973 it was shown to be a carcinogen[25]; and in 1977 it was shown to be a mutagen in *Salmonella*[15]. Its potency as a carcinogen is such that about 2 mg/kg per day in male and in female rats gives 50% of the animals cancer. (It is slightly less potent in male and female mice.) This 2 mg/kg daily level is approximately the exposure level of a worker breathing air contaminated with 2 ppm of DBCP – close to the level of actual exposure. It is too early to see if many of the workers will get cancer in 20 years, but it is not too early to see that a high percentage of them are now sterile. Currently, almost 100 workers in several companies have been made sterile or have low sperm counts as a consequence of exposures to DBCP for as little as one to two years. Because 80 industrial plants were handling the material, many more workers will probably be discovered to be similarly affected by this chemical. It is unclear how much DBCP was eaten by consumers as residues in food as there was usually no maximum level set on residues.

It seems urgent that we set up a priority list for these chemicals that have wide use and have an appreciable carcinogenic potency, and that we examine factory workers and other exposed populations for the effects of these chemicals. It seems reasonable to set human exposure limits for carcinogens on the basis of their potency and a safety factor, taking into account the chemicals' benefit to society and the alternatives.

POTENCY IN SHORT-TERM MUTAGENICITY TESTS

Although we can now make a start on human risk assessment based on animal cancer tests, few of the chemicals in the environment to which people are exposed have actually undergone cancer testing in animals. Furthermore, many of the tests that have been done lack the quality needed for making a quantitative analysis on the data. Thus we are faced with the question: can short-term tests provide any information about human risk? We are trying to answer this question, and our results so far suggest that these tests may be useful in giving an approximate idea of carcinogenic potency.

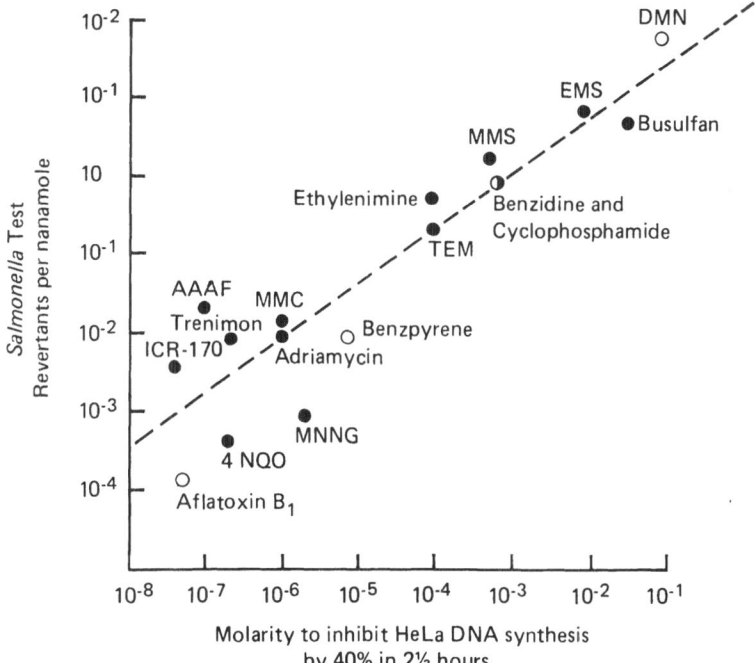

Figure 3.6   Relation between mutagenic potency of carcinogens in *Salmonella* v. potency in inhibiting DNA synthesis in the HeLa human cell line. (From R. B. Painter and R. Howard, *Mutation Res.* **54**, 113 (1978))

There is over a million-fold range in mutagenic potency in the *Salmonella* test and a similar range in carcinogenic potency. Although one would not expect a precise quantitative correlation between mutagenicity in bacteria and carcinogenicity in animals, even a rough quantitative correlation would be useful in human risk assessment. Work done by Meselson and Russell[23] suggests there is a quantitative correlation of potencies, not only for carcinogens in the same class, but also across a broad range of classes, although some nitrosamines did not fit this general relationship. Our own work (Hooper, Friedman, Sawyer, and Ames) comparing the potency of chemicals in causing tumours in rats with potency in the *Salmonella* test (using a rat liver homogenate for activation) shows a good correlation so far, with some exceptions. Additional work will show how general this correlation is. We plan to obtain *Salmonella* mutagenicity data on all those carcinogens for which we can get carcinogenic potency data. We are also examining to what extent those cases of a chemical differing in carcinogenic potency between species can be correlated with mutagenic potency assayed using the liver homogenates from the different species. Other short-term tests that are currently being developed can also be calibrated against our carcinogenic potency index to see how well they correlate. The quantitative agreement between *Salmonella* and another short-term test (inhibition of DNA synthesis in human HeLa cells in tissue culture) has been recently examined and appears good (Figure 3.6). If several short-term tests can be shown to provide rough quantitative results consistent with those from animal cancer tests, a battery of short-term tests could then be used for establishing priorities among the many mutagens, both natural and man-made, that have never been tested in animal cancer tests and to which there is significant human exposure.

DIETARY CARCINOGENS AND MUTAGENS

Man-made chemicals have been emphasized in the previous sections, and it has been pointed out that the major effect of these as carcinogens and mutagens will only become apparent in the next decades. Much of the cancer of today, on the other hand, appears to be due to cigarette smoke, radiation (e.g., ultraviolet light induces skin cancer), and the ingestion of a wide variety of natural carcinogens present in our diet. Plants have developed a wide assortment of chemicals to discourage insects and animals from eating them and many of these are mutagens and carcinogens present in the human diet[2]. In addition, powerful nitrosamine and nitrosamide carcinogens are formed from certain normal dietary biochemicals containing nitrogen, by reaction with nitrite. Nitrite is produced by bacteria in the body from nitrates that are present in ingested plant material and water[2]. A number of moulds produce powerful carcinogens such as aflatoxin and sterigmatocystin that can be present in small amounts in food contaminated by moulds, such as peanut butter and corn[2]. We discuss below the evidence that broiling food can result in the formation of considerable amounts of mutagens. *Salmonella* and the other short-term tests should play a key role as a bioassay for identifying these natural carcinogens, the first step in learning how to deal with them.

Two test cases of major importance are in progress using our *Salmonella* test as a bioassay for natural carcinogens. Dr W. R. Bruce and his colleagues in Toronto have found a considerable amount of a powerful mutagen in human faeces[2]. It appears to be a nitrosamine formed from a component of dietary fat and could be a major cause of colon and breast cancer, two common cancer types associated with high fat intake. Dr Bruce is identifying its chemical structure using *Salmonella* mutagenicity as a bioassay. He has some evidence that high vitamin C or vitamin E intake lowers the amount of the mutagen. In another instance, Dr Sugimura and his colleagues in Tokyo have discovered that when fish are broiled (a common practice in Japan), mutagenic chemicals are formed[26]. Using the *Salmonella* test as a bioassay, they have found that the broiling protein produces mutagens and that broiling tryptophan (a component of protein) produces potent mutagens. They have identified one active mutagen chemically and shown that it is also very active in another short-term assay (transformation) using animal cells. They are currently doing an animal cancer test on the substance. An animal cancer test could never have been used as the bioassay for identifying the chemical because of the time involved. Thus, based on the mutagenic activity for *Salmonella*, it appears that broiling food so that burnt protein is formed may contribute a fairly substantial dose of mutagens to our diet. Eating a barbecued fish or steak could well be equivalent to smoking a few packets of cigarettes in terms of the amount of mutagen that enters our body.

PREVENTION OF DNA DAMAGE AND PUBLIC POLICY

We believe that the problem of cancer and genetic birth defects can be usefully attacked by prevention. The following approaches are suggested.

1. *Identifying mutagens and carcinogens* from among the wide variety of environmental chemicals to which humans are exposed. All approaches

must be used: human epidemiology for cancer and genetic birth defects; animal cancer tests; and short-term mutagenicity, and transformation, tests.

2. *Pre-market testing* of new chemicals to which humans will be exposed. We have seen, and will continue to see, the folly of using people as guinea pigs.

3. *Information* could be made available on chemicals capable of causing cancer and mutations, including their relative danger where this is known, for use by government, industry, unions, consumer groups, and the public at large.

4. *Minimizing human exposure* to these chemicals, starting with those that need the most attention and working down the list. The priority list would be based on the amounts of human exposure to each chemical and the potency of the chemical in animal cancer tests. Where adequate animal cancer data are not available, potency information from *several* suitable short-term tests, such as *Salmonella*, which can be obtained quickly, might be substituted when they are validated for this purpose. The particular 'chemical of concern' at any one time may often be a mixture, such as air pollutants from auto exhaust (which is quite mutagenic in *Salmonella*). A general attack on a problem may sometimes be called for, for example, minimizing the use of mutagenic, carcinogenic, or untested chemical pesticides by education about potential hazards, product use, or alternatives, and incentives, penalties and taxes where necessary.

It seems clear that we will not be able to ban all the carcinogens and mutagens because too many exist and many are of great economic importance. Thus, setting priorities and trying to minimize human exposure are essential. The carcinogen and mutagen vinyl chloride is still used in the plastics industry to make vinyl floor tiles and PVC pipe, but vinyl chloride is no longer used in millions of cosmetic spray cans, and workers are no longer breathing in a dose that could give a high percentage of them cancer.

References

1. Doll, R. (1977). 'Strategy for detection of cancer hazards to man', *Nature (London)*, **265 (5595)**, 589
2. Hiatt, H. H. Watson, J. D. and Winsten, J. A. (eds.). (1977). *Origins of Human Cancer*, Vol. 4, books A, B, C, Cold Spring Harbor Conferences on Cell Proliferation. (Cold Spring Harbor, New York: Cold Spring Harbor Laboratory, 1977)
3. Fishbein, L. (1977). *Potential Industrial Carcinogens and Mutagens*. U.S. Environmental Protection Agency, **560/5-77-005**

4. Maugh, T. H. II. (1978). 'Chemicals: How many are there?' *Science*, **199** (4325), 162
5. Rapoport, I. A. (1961). 'The reaction of genic proteins with 1,2-dichloro-ethane', *Translation of Doklady Biological Sciences Sections* (*Doklady Akademii Nauk SSSR*), **134** (1–6), trans. of *Dokl. Akad. Nauk SSSR* (1960). **134 (5)**
6. Shakarnis, V. F. (1969). '1,2 Dichloroethane-induced chromosome non-disjunction and recessive sex-linked lethal mutation in *Drosophila melanogaster*', *Genetika* (USSR), **5 (12)**, 89
7. Carter, L. J. (1976). 'Michigan's PBB incident: Chemical mix-up leads to disaster', *Science*, **192 (4326)**, 240
8. Dougherty, R. C. and Piotrowska, K. (1976). 'Screening by negative chemical ionization mass spectrometry for environmental contamination with toxic residues: Application to human urine', *Proc. Natl. Acad. Sci. USA*, **73 (6)**, 1777
9. Krotoszynski, B. Gabriel, G. O'Neill, H. and Claudio, M. P. A. (1977). 'Characterization of human expired air: A promising investigative and diagnostic technique', *J. Chromatog. Sci.*, **15 (7)**, 239
10. Crump, K. S., Hoel, D. G., Langley, C. H. and Peto, R. (1976). 'Fundamental carcinogenic processes and their implications for low dose risk assessment', *Cancer Res.*, **36 (9)**, 2973
11. Guess, H. Crump, K. and Peto, R. (1977). 'Uncertainty estimates for low-dose-rate extrapolations of animal carcinogenicity data', *Cancer Res.*, **37 (10)**, 3475
12. Ames, B. N., McCann, J. and Yamasaki, E. (1975). 'Methods for detecting carcinogens and mutagens with the *Salmonella*/mammalian–microsome mutagenicity test', *Mutat. Res.*, **31 (6)**, 347
13. McCann, J., Choi, E., Yamasaki, E. and Ames, B. N. (1975). 'Detection of carcinogens as mutagens in the *Salmonella*/microsome test: Assay of 300 chemicals', *Proc. Natl. Acad. Sci. USA*, **72 (12)**, 5135
14. McCann, J. and Ames, B. N. (1976). 'Detection of carcinogens as mutagens in the *Salmonella*/microsome test: Assay of 300 chemicals: Discussion', *Proc. Natl. Acad. Sci. USA*, **73 (3)**, 950
15. McCann, J. and Ames, B. N. (1977). 'The *Salmonella*/microsome mutagenicity test: Predictive values for animal carcinogenicity', In H. H. Hiatt, J. D. Watson and J. A. Winsten (eds.). *Origins of Human Cancer*, vol. 4, book C, pp. 1431–1450
16. Sugimura, T. *et al.* (1977). 'Mutagen-carcinogens in food, with special reference to highly mutagenic pyrolytic products in broiled foods', In H. H. Hiatt, J. D. Watson and J. A. Winsten (eds.). *Origins of Human Cancer*, vol. 4, book C, pp. 1561–1577
17. Inui, N., Nishi, Y. and Taketomi, M. (1978). 'Mutagenic effect of orally given AF-2 on embryonic cells in pregnant Syrian hamsters', *Mutat. Res.*, **57 (1)**, 69
18. Blum, A. and Ames, B. N. (1977). 'Flame-retardant additives as possible cancer hazards'. *Science*, **195 (4273)**, 17
19. Prival, M. J., McCoy, E. C., Gutter, B. and Rosenkranz, H. S. (1977). 'Tris (2,3-dibromopropyl)phosphate: Mutagenicity of a widely used flame retardant', *Science*, **195 (4273)**, 76

20. Ames, B. N., Kammen, H. O. and Yamasaki, E. (1975). 'Hair dyes are mutagenic: Identification of a variety of mutagenic ingredients', *Proc. Natl. Acad. Sci. USA*, **72 (6)**, 2423

21. Kier, L. D., Yamasaki, E. and Ames, B. N. (1974). 'Detection of mutagenic activity in cigarette smoke condensates', *Proc. Natl. Acad. Sci. USA*, **71 (10)**, 4159

22. Yamasaki, E. and Ames, B. N. (1977). 'Concentration of mutagens from urine by absorption with the nonpolar resin XAD-2: Cigarette smokers have mutagenic urine', *Proc. Natl. Acad. USA*, **74 (8)**, 3555–3559

23. Meselson, M. and Russell, K. (1977). 'Comparisons of carcinogenic and mutagenic potency', In H. H. Hiatt, J. D. Watson and J. A. Winston (eds.). *Origins of Human Cancer*, vol. 4, book C, pp. 1473–1481

24. Torkelson, T. R., Sadek, S. E., Rowe, V. K., Kodama, J. K. Anderson, H. H., Loquvam, G. S. and Hine, C. H. (1961). 'Toxicologic investigations of 1,2-dibromo-3-chloropropane', *Toxicolog. App. Pharmacol.*, **3 (5)**, 545–559

25. Olson, W. A., Huberman, R. T., Weisburger, E. K., Word, J. M. and Weisburger, J. H. (1973). 'Induction of stomach cancer in rats and mice by halogenated aliphatic fumigants', *J. Natl. Cancer Inst.*, **51 (6)**, 1993

26. Nagao, M. *et al.* (1977). 'Mutagens in foods, and especially pyrolysis products of protein', In D. Scott, B. A. Bridges, and F. H. Sobels (eds.). *Progress in Genetic Toxicology* (Amsterdam: Elsevier/North Holland)

4

Practical experience in
testing unknowns *in vitro*
D. B. McGregor

Since the early years of this decade, many laboratories have used to advantage a test which has been repeatedly described as a very sensitive and simple bacterial test for detecting chemical mutagens and is now generally called Ames' test[1]. This test has been used in our laboratories since 1973 and it is from this use that I shall draw examples of practical experience in testing unknowns *in vitro*. For this clear restriction I make no apology because, in specializing more time can be given to demonstrating that while the test is indeed simple in execution and sensitive in its powers to detect chemical mutagens problems of interpretation can arise. The interpretative problems described are not necessarily confined to Ames' test since they are also met with in other *in vitro* mutation tests.

IS THE COMPOUND A MUTAGEN?

A crucial factor in the testing for mutagenic activity of previously untested substances is the need for criteria to demonstrate that a negative response is a reasonable basis for concluding that a substance is indeed non-mutagenic in the assay. Equally fundamental is the need to demonstrate that an apparently positive response is a reasonable basis for concluding that a substance is truly mutagenic.

If a chemical is tested adequately and fails to produce a doubling of the spontaneous mutation frequency at some dose level, then it is defined as not being a mutagen detectable in Ames' test. Should a doubling of the spontaneous frequency be observed, then a dose–response should also be demonstrable in order to confirm the suspected mutagenic effect. This commonly held pragmatic concept has been discussed on statistical grounds by Ehrenberg who concludes in specific examples that the beta-error (i.e. the observed probability that not rejecting a hypothesis is incorrect) is satisfactorily small, even when it is recognized that spontaneous control values do vary from experiment to experiment[2]. This doubling concept is not followed in some laboratories where something less than a doubling of the spontaneous mutation frequency (or numbers of mutants per plate) is accepted if there is a dose–related trend. There can be no quarrel with this attitude if this dose–related trend is reproducible.

The major point is the criteria for *adequate* testing. These criteria may be listed as follows:

1. The test organisms have preserved their identity and have not lost their ability to respond to specific, known mutagens.

2. The activation system is of an acceptable standard as shown, for example, by the activity of selected foreign compound metabolizing enzymes and by the formation of mutagenic metabolites from known pro-mutagens.

3. All other general aspects of the test system are properly quality controlled.

4. The test compound is in close contact with the bacteria at adequate concentrations.

Each of these points will be dealt with in turn.

Test organism authentication

Methods for identification of the test organisms have been well described in various publications[1,3] and will not be detailed here, apart from a single aspect (Table 4.1). *Salmonella typhimurium* strain TA 100 is derived from strain TA 1535, which is a base-pair substitution indicator strain. In addition to the TA 1535 genome, TA 100 contains a plasmid, pKM101, which is an incomplete form of the plasmid R46. The properties of these plasmids have been studied in some detail by Walker[4] and by Mortelmans and Stocker[5].

The plasmid pKM101 causes the bacteria to be more sensitive to certain mutagens. It also causes the bacterium to be resistant to ampicillin and to have a high spontaneous mutation frequency. Colony counts of around

Table 4.1   Possible *S. typhimurium* **culture batch identification procedure**

Criterion	TA 1535	TA 1537	TA 1538	TA 98	TA 100
Crystal violet sensitive	+	+	+	+	+
Ampicillin sensitive	+	+	+	−	−
Mutated by:					
9-aminoacridine		+			
2-nitrofluorene			+	+	
sodium azide	+				+

140 per plate are considered normal for TA 100, although considerable variation does occur. For example, Brown *et al.*[6] quote as historical control values 94 $\pm$ 25 without activation and 87 $\pm$ 24 with activation on 205 and 192 plates respectively.

In scientific publications, spontaneous counts greater than 300 have been quoted and low counts are also encountered. From time to time we have experienced TA 100 counts as low as 35–40 per plate and on rare occasions the counts have been indistinguishable from those of TA 1535, yet ampicillin resistance remains[7]. This resistance is an important marker and is usually demonstrated in our laboratory by spreading the bacteria on non-specific medium and placing a 2 μg ampicillin disc in the centre of the plate, which is then incubated overnight. The absence of a zone of inhibition confirms the identity of TA 100. Should the plasmid be lost then the zone of inhibition will appear as it does in TA 1535. With TA 1535, for example, there is a completely clear zone about 5 mm wide around the 2 μg ampicillin disc. Recently, we have decided to use 10 μg discs instead. This is because cultures with low spontaneous colony counts show *partial* inhibition to 10 μg ampicillin discs manifest as a zone with some clearing of the normal lawn of microcolonies. This effect is interesting and deserves investigation since this zone is not seen with the 2 μg disc which, nevertheless, totally inhibits TA 1535 growth. A mixed culture of authentic TA 1535 and TA 100 would be expected to show partial growth inhibition even with the 2 μg ampicillin disc.

Another interesting observation is that strain TA 100 cultures with low spontaneous colony counts are still sensitive to an undiminished degree to chemical mutagens which are detected by TA 100, but not by TA 1535. Chromate is one such example. The nitrofuran derivative, AF-2, is another (Figure 4.1). It appears, therefore, that provided some ampicillin resistance is observed, TA 100 cultures should be acceptable for use in mutation experiments although they may have low spontaneous mutation frequencies. It could be that there has been partial loss of plasmid in such cases – either complete copies from multiply-infected bacteria or partial structure

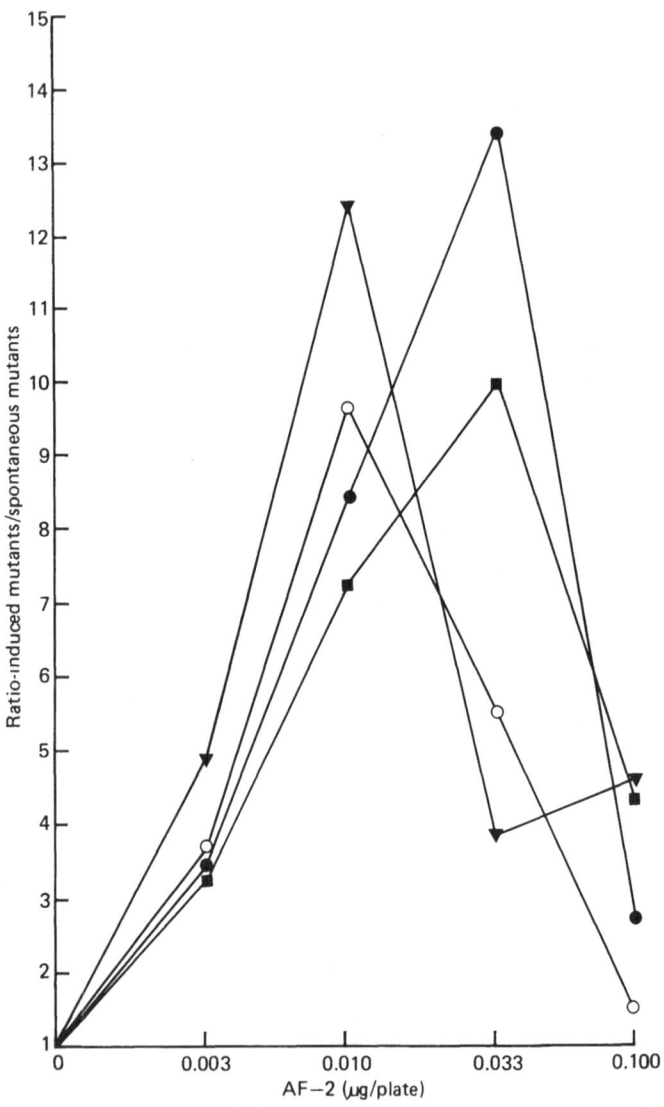

Figure 4.1   Ratios of induced to spontaneously occurred numbers of mutants obtained when four cultures of *S. typhimurium* TA 100 were treated with the nitrofuran derivative AF-2. A TA 1535 culture would show no response to AF-2. Spontaneous mutants per plate were: ▼ = 43, ○ = 41, ● = 111, ■ = 124

loss from the already incomplete R46-derived plasmid – giving reduced spontaneous mutant colony counts. The latter possibility is unlikely because the pKM101 plasmid does seem to be stable (Mortelmans, personal communication).

The hypothesis that some copies of the non-integrated plasmid are lost from the bacteria presupposes that the donated characters, such as ampicillin resistance, are gene dose dependent. This is a testable hypothesis which is presently under investigation along with a third possible explanation which is that there has been complete loss of entire copies from a proportion of the bacteria in the cultures.

In spite of this argument for the acceptability of data using low spontaneous mutation frequency TA 100 strain cultures, it may be safer to use cultures which normally provide well in excess of 100 colonies per plate unless adequate controls are performed. There is a danger also, however, in the too ready acceptance of this purely numerical criterion since there may be, rarely, a culture of low count TA 100 strain contaminated with TA 100 revertants.

Adequacy of metabolic activation system

The use of positive control substances is commonplace in *in vitro* toxicology. They are thought to give assurance that the experiment has been performed in a satisfactory manner. Their use also means that the experimenters are repeatedly and frequently exposed to substances which are known to be hazardous. If the experimenters are to expose themselves to such known, hazardous chemicals, then these chemicals must be contained, used to minimal extents and used in such a manner that the optimal effect is obtained. In Ames' tests, positive control substances may be used in characterization of the organisms: 2-nitrofluorene for TA 1538 and TA 98, daunomycin for TA 98, 9-aminoacridine for TA 1537, etc. A very useful control substance is 2-aminoanthracene which requires metabolic activation and is a mutagen detectable with the five commonly used *S. typhimurium* strains. It is unfortunate, however, that some laboratories use such unnecessarily high dose levels of this and other positive control substances. The dose–response curve with 2-aminoanthracene, for example, reaches a plateau response at a dose somewhat higher than 3 μg per plate (Figure 4.2), therefore, any dose higher than about 3 μg per plate could be misleading.

It has been our philosophy that doses close to the lowest effective dose level normally detectable should be used. If a non-significant increase in the number of mutants obtained arises from the use of such a dose level then the experiment is rejected. It has been argued that, at very low dose levels, non-significant results will be encountered in a random manner.

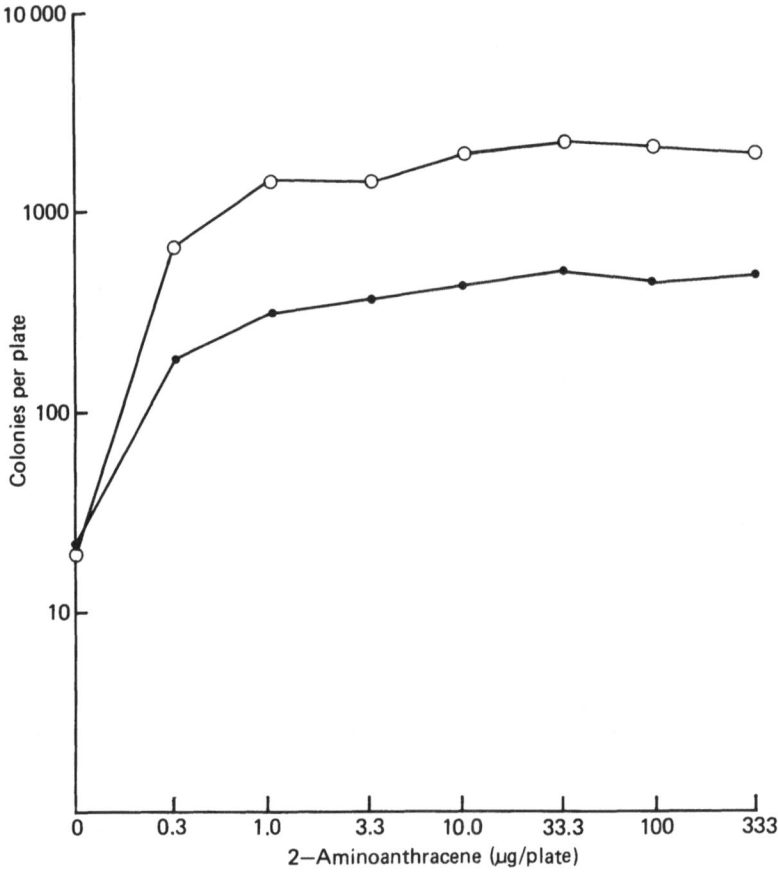

Figure 4.2 Dose–response curves with 2-aminoanthracene, using *S. typhimurium* strains TA 1535 (●) and TA 1538 (○) in the presence of non-induced rat liver S-9 mix

While this is certainly true it must also be recognized that a non-significant response may result from suboptimal reaction conditions. A non-significant response with a previously untested substance in parallel with a non-significant response with low doses of the positive control substance could mean that the previously untested substance is a weak mutagen, but suboptimal reaction conditions did not allow its detection. When higher dose levels of a positive control substance are used then the sensitivity of the reaction may not be monitored adequately. Hence, the significance of 'non-mutagenic' responses in these circumstances must be in doubt. The worst possible situation is where the response of a positive control substance requiring metabolic activation is on a plateau of the curve.

One factor limiting the response must be concentration* in the reaction medium of the ultimate mutagenic metabolite. The fact that a plateau exists at all suggests that there is a rate limiting reaction which is saturated or that, in Ames' test, there is a particularly unstable enzyme (Figure 4.3). In such a situation, measuring the product of the overall series of

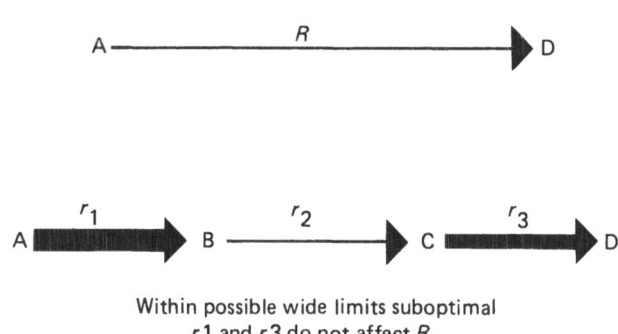

Within possible wide limits suboptimal
$r1$ and $r3$ do not affect R

Figure 4.3   Rate-limiting reactions

reactions can give no indication of suboptimal activity in a member of that series other than in the normally rate-limiting step (or, in Ames' test, the dose-limiting step).

There is, however, a problem even when the positive control response is on the ascending portion of the dose–response curve: there will be variations, but the information is not generally available to tell us what variation is acceptable.

System quality control

It has been found that certain components of the Vogel–Bonner agar plates can affect the mutation frequency obtained. If large batches of plates are to be used it is advisable to test each batch to be sure that there are not mutagens already in the plates which, of course, will increase the background frequency, possibly to unacceptable levels. Ethylene oxide or its residues may be responsible for these increases, but not necessarily so. The plates we use are not ethylene oxide sterilized yet occasionally high

* In Ames' tests it is actually the dose (= concentration × time) of the ultimate metabolite which is the limiting factor.

counts have been obtained, particularly with frameshift indicator strains. At least as disturbing was a finding in a few recent batches of plates that the positive control responses from frameshift indicator strains could be seriously reduced. A component of the medium has been implicated, but not yet identified. Such experiences dictate that batches of plates be quality controlled not only for microbial contaminants, bubbles, uneven agar distribution and so on, but also for plate effects on spontaneous and induced mutation frequencies.

Testing to system limits

It is well known that reverse mutations, such as must occur in the *S. typhimurium* strains before a mutagenic effect is detected, are indicator strain specific, e.g. 9-aminoacridine is specific for the mutation carried by TA 1537. For this reason, a battery of strains is required for testing. However, even so-called non-selective indicator systems – forward mutations in bacteria or mammalian cells, gene conversion in yeasts – do have an element of selectivity. It is, then, necessary to test a substance to the limits of the system used to be sure that it is *not* inducing an observable effect simply because none of the commonly recognized indicator strains is readily reverted by the type of mutation that substance induces.

The limits imposed by the system are test compound solubility and indicator organism survival. Without the demonstration at some dose level of either or both of these limits with a variety of indicator organisms, a negative result must always be viewed with suspicion.

Certain chemicals induce mutations above the background frequency over a relatively narrow dose range. Early in our use of the test we would use 5-fold steps in our dose range, e.g. 5 μg, 25 μg, 125 μg, etc. The use of such steps led to the necessity for many repetitions of tests, however, and half-log steps are now routinely used, e.g. 3.3 μg, 10 μg, 33 μg, etc.

In this way, dose–responses are more often demonstrated in the first experiment with a mutagenic substance and there is less possibility of not recognizing a mutagen because the mutagenic 'window' was totally or partially missed.

Special problems are posed by volatile chemicals, so various devices have been used to overcome them. Low boiling point liquids, for example, can be fed through calibrated rotameters to give the required atmospheric concentration (Figure 4.4). Perhaps the least satisfactory situation exists with liquids which have appreciable partial pressures at around 37 °C. The rotameter device is not suitable for them and they cannot be tested in an open system because they will evaporate from the plates. To deal with

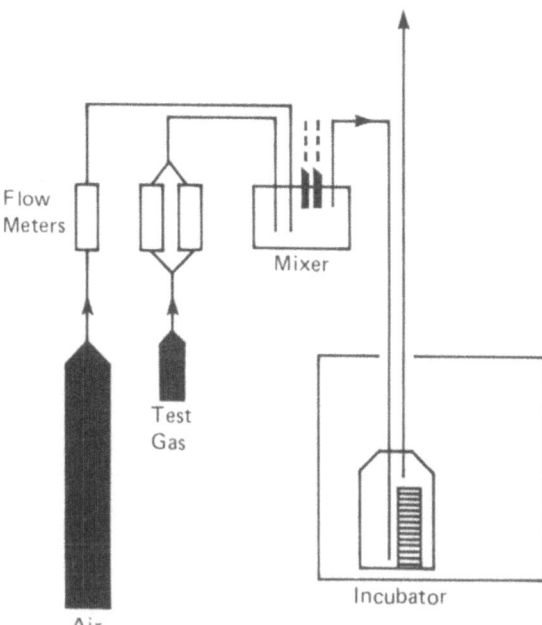

Figure 4.4 Scheme by which metered flow rates of test gas and air can be mixed and distributed to different exposure chambers. This system has been used with arctons (freons)

these substances we incubate our plates in an enclosed vessel (Figure 4.5). The free air space of the vessel containing plates is measured and a calculated quantity of test substance weighed into a tube which is then frozen in liquid nitrogen for some minutes. The tube is rapidly transferred to the exposure chamber which is sealed and partially evacuated. Following incubation at 37 °C for about 2 h, air is admitted to return the chamber to ambient pressure. In this way, it is hoped that the atmospheric concentration will be known and test substance kept in contact with the bacteria.

PITFALLS IN RESULT INTERPRETATION

It is very easy to make wrong assumptions about a test and the results it yields unless vigilance is maintained. For this reason I am emphatic in my belief that this simple test should be performed in such a way that the routine experimenters remain involved – they should not be working at a result assembly line – and the tests should not be turned over to cheap

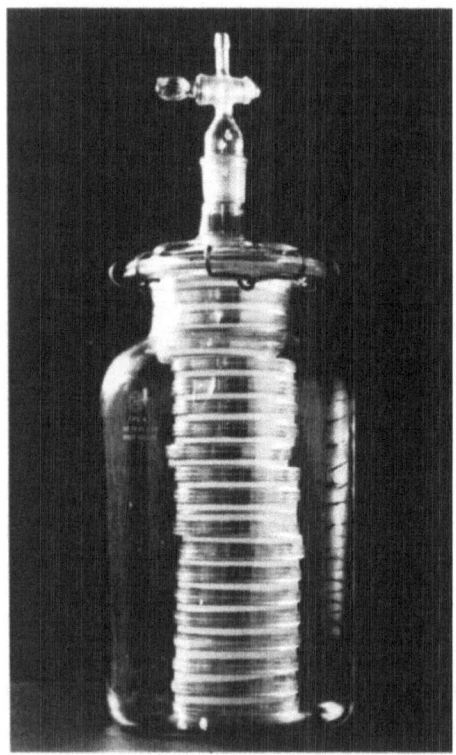

Figure 4.5 Exposure chamber for testing substances with high partial pressures at 37°C

labour with no background in a relevant science. Some pitfalls encountered in experimentation will now be described.

Dichloromethane

Dichloromethane boils at 39 °C, so it is treated as a volatile liquid requiring containment with the indicator organism during testing. Theoretical atmospheric concentrations of dichloromethane under the test conditions of temperature and pressure are easily calculated.

It is important to point out, however, that the actual atmospheric concentration may be very different from what was calculated.

Dichloromethane has been shown to be a mutagen in *S. typhimurium* in several laboratories. We have tested several different samples supplied

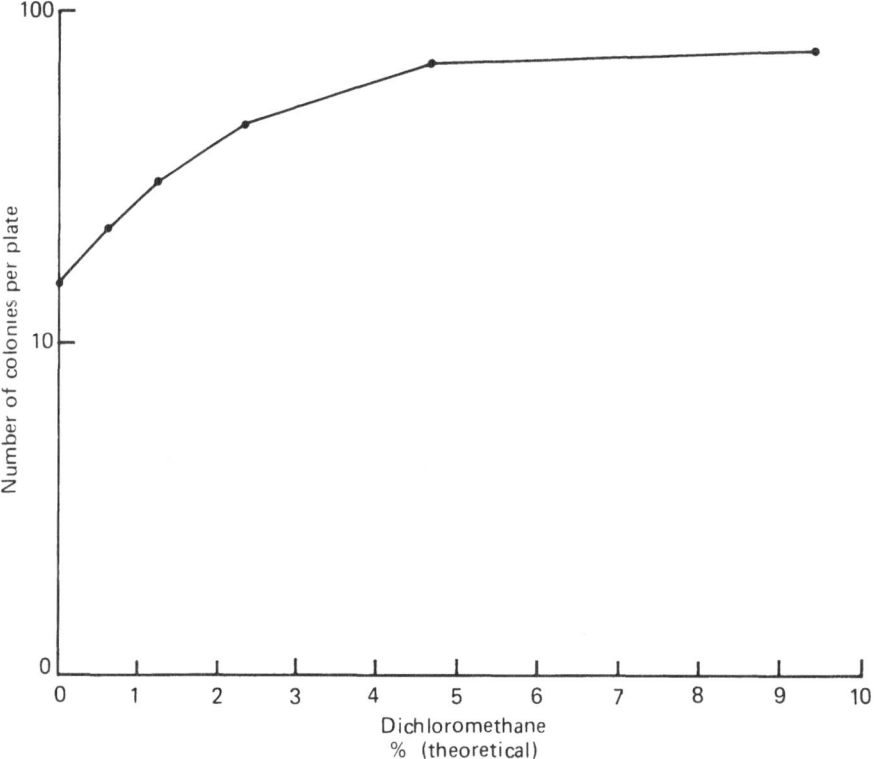

Figure 4.6 Dose–response curve obtained when *S. typhimurium* TA 1535 was treated with dichloromethane

over several years and can confirm this result with strains TA 100 and, to a lesser extent, TA 1535 (Figure 4.6). The results have been published only recently[8].

In our experiments the actual atmospheric concentrations were monitored by gas chromatography on a glass column filled with 10 % OV101 on Chromasorb W80–100 mesh. Actual quantities of dichloromethane on the agar plates were also measured using a headspace – gas chromatography analytical method (Table 4.2).

Actual atmospheric concentrations were only approximately half the theoretical values based on the weights of dichloromethane used, but the quantities dissolved in the agar, or condensed on its surface, did increase in relation to the atmospheric concentrations.

Certain possible reasons for the discrepancy between theoretical and actual atmospheric concentrations were checked.

Table 4.2   Dichloromethane concentrations. Calculated and measured concentrations differ by a factor of
approximately × 3 in the atmosphere. Condensation
on to the agar and solution in the water accounts for
some of the discrepancy

| Atmospheric | | Total per plate | |
Theoretical	Actual		
0	nd		nd
0.5%	0.14%		245 μg
1.0%	0.33%	(1)	600 μg
		(2)	595 μg
		(3)	530 μg
2.0%	0.67%		1400 μg
4.0%	1.60%		2425 μg

nd   Not detected

1. There was no significant loss of dichloromethane during partial evacuation of the exposure chamber.

2. Visual inspection showed that no liquid dichloromethane remained in the sample tube after warming the exposure chamber to 37 °C.

3. Minimal quantities of silicone grease were used on the stockcock of the exposure chamber and it is considered unlikely that significant quantities of dichloromethane would be absorbed by the grease.

4. Non-linearity of the flame ionization detector response, in the gas chromatograph, to chlorinated molecules is well known, therefore, chromatography was conducted at an attenuation where linearity of response had been established.

The reason for the discrepancy in atmospheric concentrations has not been established, but it does exist, is reproducible and occurs even when glass petri dishes are used in the experiment. Plastic petri dishes, as normally used, could absorb dichloromethane to an appreciable degree. Perhaps the most likely explanation is that there has been condensation on to the walls of the exposure chamber. Unfortunately, this is a very difficult proposal to verify directly. This discrepancy is being stressed because there may be a temptation in the industrial environment to make value judgements on the significance of mutagenic effects at atmospheric concentrations which are not, perhaps, what they are supposed to be. Also, it is as well to realize that the dose to the bacteria must depend upon the partitioning of the test substance between air and water. It can be expected that the effective dose to bacteria will be high with a substance which tends to condense and dissolve in water. On the other hand the effective dose will be low with volatile, hydrophobic substances which may be, nevertheless, rather readily transported across oily human skin.

Paraquat

A dose–response does not always have a positive sign, maxima in plotted curves often being seen. Possible reasons for such curves are, for example:

1. Toxicity of the test substance to the test organism.
2. Specific toxicity of the test substance to the revertants.
3. In those cases where metabolic activation is required the test substance may inhibit the liver enzymes involved in the reactions. Extreme evidence for this last effect has been observed where, at high doses, the postmitochondrial supernatant has precipitated yet the bacteria grow to a satisfactory degree.

A chemical with a specific effect against revertants could be an inhibitor of amino acid or protein synthesis, but not necessarily. For example, paraquat is a chemical which, at moderate dose levels, caused a reduction to or close to zero of the number of mutants per plate (Figure 4.7). There was a lawn of microcolonies on these plates which appeared to be normal. At yet higher dose levels, there was thinning of the background lawn, which is indicative of toxicity, and some microcolonies grew to a size where they were observable without the aid of a microscope. My colleague, Malcolm McConville, postulated that there might be differential toxicity of paraquat for his^- and his^+ bacteria. This would explain the observation that the mutants spontaneously occurring disappeared from the plates before the lawn of microcolonies thinned. He tested his hypothesis by taking spontaneous revertants (his^+) and countable colonies from some high-dose paraquat plates and growing them on nutrient agar plates with a central well containing a standard quantity of paraquat. By measuring the area of the clear zone around the well, following incubation, the sensitivities of the various cultures could be compared (Table 4.3). The spontaneous revertants were found to be more sensitive to the toxicity of paraquat than the colonies recovered from high-dose paraquat plates. Furthermore, very few of these colonies were his^+, i.e. they were not mutants. Hence, it was concluded that in spite of the increase in the number of colonies at high doses of paraquat, this herbicide is not mutagenic in *S. typhimurium* in Ames' test.

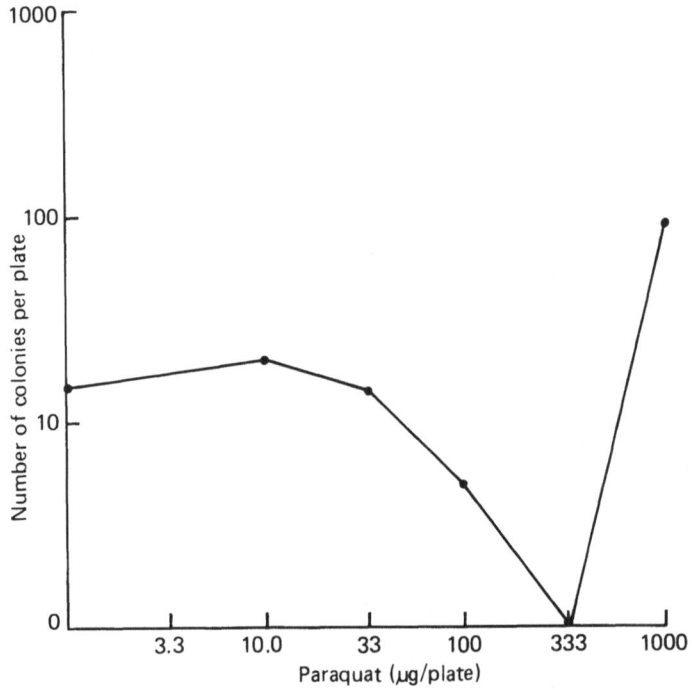

Figure 4.7   The effect of paraquat on the number of colonies per plate obtained
with *S. typhimurium* TA 98. The increase seen at high dose levels is not due to
mutants

**Table 4.3   Resistance to paraquat of *S.
typhimurium* TA 98. Relative growth inhibition of large colonies from 5 mg paraquat
dose plate***

TA 98 (parental)	100%
TA 98/Pq 20	59%
TA 98/Pq 39	59%
TA 98/Pq 46	56%
TA 98/Pq 63	62%
TA 98/Pq 84	59%

* Only 2/102 isolates were his$^+$

Benzil

It is known from mammalian cell culture work that photoreaction products
formed in media stored in fluorescent or natural light are toxic to cells. In
addition to the possibility that such light-generated products are also

mutagenic, white light itself is known to induce mutations in mammalian cells. Also, radicals are frequently produced by white light and many of the solvents commonly used act as 'sensitizers' in photochemical reactions. It is, therefore, possible that differing lighting conditions can contribute to interlaboratory discrepancies in results. A clear example of this came to our notice a few months ago when benzil was tested under our normal laboratory lighting conditions, which are white light during the brief time required for weighing and dilution of the test compound and amber light or darkness for the remainder of the experiment. Benzil was found to be very weakly mutagenic, whereas in another laboratory a strong response was obtained. Light was one factor differing in the two laboratories, therefore, the experiment was repeated in our laboratory, some plates being deliberately exposed to sunlight at a window for 15 min after the bacteria and benzil had been mixed and poured on them under amber light. Lids were left in place on all plates after pouring, so, ultraviolet light was not responsible for any effect seen. While no mutagenic response was seen with plates exposed only to amber light, a significant response was observed on the natural light-exposed plates (Figure 4.8). It is not known whether the mutagenic effect is due to radicals or oxidation products from radical reactions.

Following this experience with benzil, it has recently been shown[9] that benzo(a)pyrene is mutagenic without metabolic activation in some of the *Salmonella* strains if it is first irradiated. The radiation sources used were ^{60}Co, an ultraviolet germicidal lamp and a white fluorescent striplight. All sources were effective in producing mutagenic products from benzo(a) pyrene in the dry state. Exposure to the striplight was for 18 days on Whatman No. 1 filter paper. While non-exposed benzo(a)pyrene recovered from the paper was, as expected, non-mutagenic, the recovered light-exposed material induced highly significant increases in the numbers of mutants. The photo-oxidation products supposed to be responsible for the mutagenic activity have not been identified. It would be interesting to discover whether short exposures to white light of oxygenated benzo(a) pyrene *solutions* had similar effects. Perhaps unstable radicals are formed which can damage DNA if their formation occurs in the close proximity of the bacteria. Single electron reactions have been postulated as a mechanism by which electrophilic products are generated *in vivo* and *in vitro* from benzo(a)pyrene[10]. A very preliminary experiment along these lines has been conducted in our laboratory. The benzo(a)pyrene was dissolved in DMSO and either kept in the dark or exposed to natural light (diffuse sunlight) in daytime for one day.

Test plates were prepared in amber light with these solutions which were

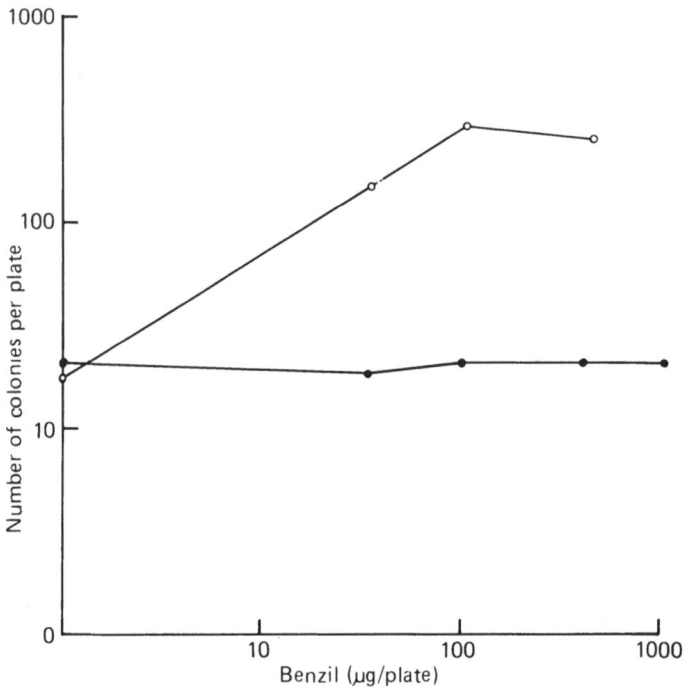

Figure 4.8 Effect of short exposure of plates to diffuse sunlight when *S. typhimurium* TA 1538 is treated with benzil: ● experiment wholly in amber light; ○ experiment with 15 min exposure of plates to sunlight

then either kept in the dark or exposed to diffuse sunlight for one hour. The plates were then incubated for three days. Where neither benzo(a) pyrene solution nor plates were exposed to white light there was no toxicity or mutagenicity (in the absence of liver preparations) with any dose level up to 333 μg per plate, at which dose precipitation occurred. Exposure of benzo(a)pyrene solution to natural light resulted in the production of a so-called direct-acting mutagen, thereby supplementing the results of Gibson *et al.*[9]. If, however, plates with either light-exposed or non-exposed benzo(a)pyrene solutions were light-exposed for 1 h toxic substances were generated which killed bacteria even at a dose of only 33 μg per plate.

These preliminary experiments suggest several new lines of investigation, but they immediately show the importance of detailed description of experimental conditions which may influence the results in unexpected ways. Considering the specific influence of light, it is possible that, in an experiment conducted in white light, toxic substances may be produced at dose levels below those required to demonstrate a mutagenic effect. Alternatively, as in the experiments of Gibson *et al.*[9], substances normally considered non-mutagenic and non-carcinogenic, such as pyrene and fluorene, may be oxidized through single electron reactions to mutagenic products.

COLOURANT COMPONENTS

Several laboratories have become involved with the testing of food and hair colourants, many of which are mutagenic. Dye manufacture often depends on long-used traditional processes and the product is by no means pure. The presence of appreciable quantities of impurities inevitably raises the question of the importance of such impurities to the resulting mutagenic effect.

Figure 4.9 shows the small but significant differences seen in the mutagenic effects of a food colourant used in certain countries. The colourant

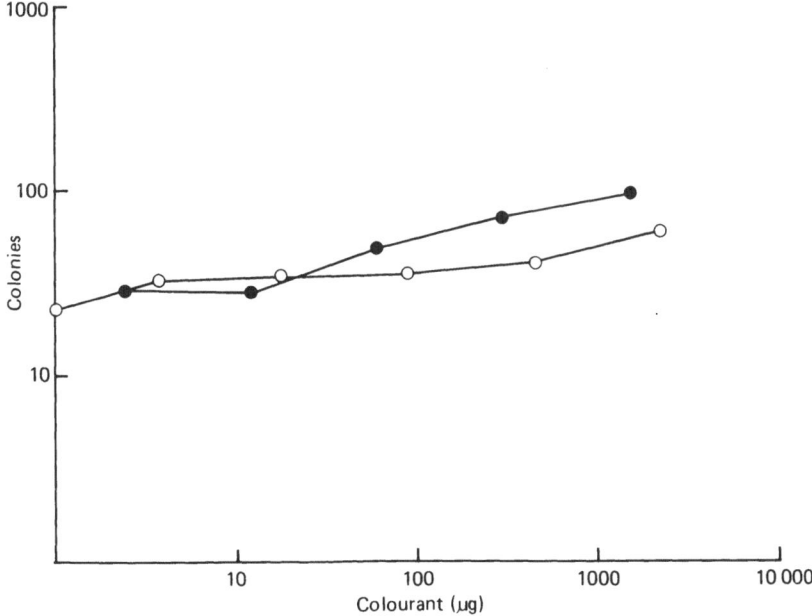

Figure 4.9 Effects of nominally the same food colourant from two separate manufacturers on the mutation frequency of *S. typhimurium* TA 1538

was tested as supplied from two independent manufacturers. Even more obvious, however, is the difference in mutagenic potential of nominally the same hair colourant obtained from two manufacturers (Figure 4.10). Results such as these demonstrate the importance of checking supply sources for differences in manufacturing processes and for giving consideration to cleaning up ingredients in order to reduce or, hopefully, even abolish a mutagenic effect seen in the crude product.

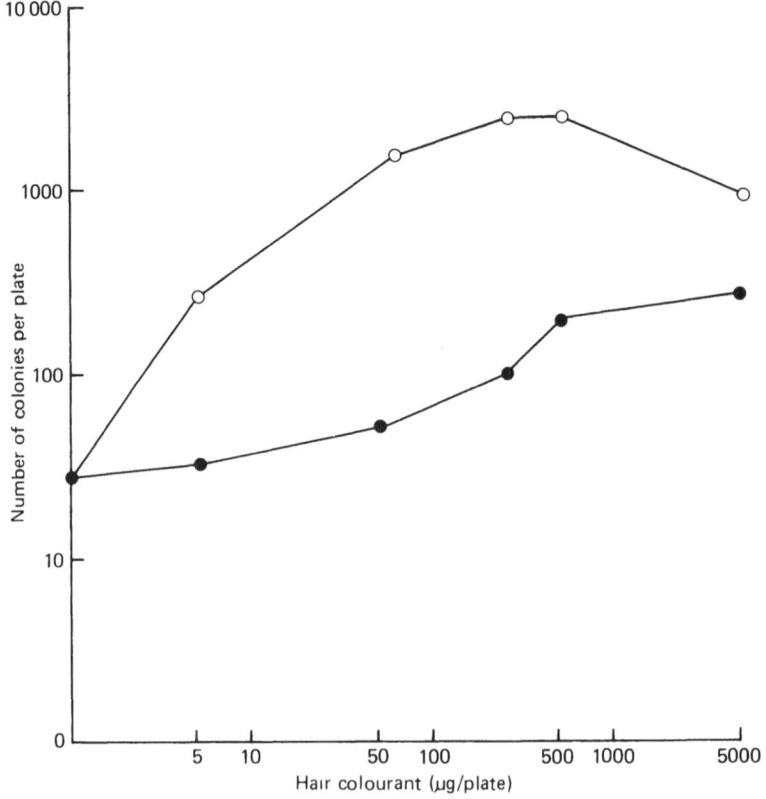

Figure 4.10 Effects of nominally the same hair colourant from two separate manufacturers on the mutation frequency of *S. typhimurium* TA 98

CONCLUSION

Further examples of experiments illustrating different experiences could easily be found, for example the difficulties of testing microbial enzyme preparations for use as food additives; the interpretation of results with substances mutagenic without metabolic activation, but not mutagenic in the presence of liver preparations; the exposure time effect seen with several halogenated hydrocarbons[7]; the problems associated with setting up reaction conditions in order to test unstable intermediates formed in industrial processes; and so on. Examples of these points can be found in the scientific journals and this chapter only serves to draw attention to the variety of problems which can be encountered.

References

1. Ames, B. N., Lee, F. D. and Durston, W. E. (1973). An improved bacterial test system for the detection and classification of mutagens and carcinogens. *Proc. Nat. Acad. Sci. USA* **70**, 782
2. Ehrenberg, L. (1971). Aspects of statistical inference in testing for genetic toxicity. In B. J. Kilbey, M. Legator, W. Nichols and C. Ramel (eds.). *Handbook of Mutagenicity Test Procedures*, Elsevier/North-Holland Biomedical Press, Amsterdam.
3. Ames, B. N., McCann, J. and Yamasaki, E. (1975). Methods for detecting carcinogens and mutagens with the *Salmonella*/mammalian-microsome mutagenicity test. *Mutat. Res.*, **31**, 347
4. Walker, G. C. (1978). Isolation and characterization of mutants of the plasmid pKM101 deficient in their ability to enhance mutagenesis and repair. *J. Bacteriol.*, **133**, 1203
5. Mortelmans, K. E. and Stocker, B. A. D. (1978). Segregation of the mutator property of plasmid R46 from its ultraviolet-protecting property. *Molec. Gen. Genet.* (Accepted for publication.)
6. Brown, J. P., Roehm, G. W. and Brown, R. J. (1978). Mutagenicity testing of certified food colors and related azo, xanthene and triphenylmethane dyes with the *Salmonella*/microsome system. *Mutat. Res.*, **56**, 249
7. Longstaff, E. and McGregor, D. B. (1978). Mutagenicity of a halocarbon refrigerant monochlorodifluoromethane (R-22) in *Salmonella typhimurium*. *Toxicol. Lett.*, **2**, 1
8. Jongen, W. M. F., Alink, G. M. and Koeman, J. H. (1978). Mutagenic effect of dichloromethane on *S. typhimurium*. *Mutat. Res.*, **56**, 245
9. Gibson, T. L., Smart, V. B. and Smith, L. L. (1978). Non-enzymic activation of polycyclic hydrocarbons as mutagens. *Mutat. Res.*, **49**, 153
10. Ts'o, P.O.P., Caspary, W. J., Leavitt, J. C., Lesko, S. A. and Lorentzen, R. J. (1976). One-electron oxidation of benzo(a)pyrene in chemical and metabolic processes. In '*In vitro* Metabolic Activation in Mutagenesis Testing', F. J. de Serres, J. R. Fouts, J. R., Bend and R. M. Philpot North-Holland Biomedical Press (Elsevier/Amsterdam)

5

Induced mutation in micro-organisms: validity for estimating risk to man

L. Ehrenberg

It is generally agreed that a compound clearly demonstrated to induce mutation in micro-organisms should be considered a potential risk to man, and, as beautifully formulated in Bridges' three-tier system[1], if exposure to the compound would be advantageous to human health, wellbeing or economy, a quantitation of risks to man has to be introduced into the cost–benefit evaluation. If a test is negative, and if the compound is important, it has to be questioned whether the test is qualitatively reliable and, if so, whether it is sensitive enough to detect an unacceptable risk. The same reasoning is required in the case of physical agents such as electromagnetic fields.

Risks of heritable damage and cancer in human beings exposed to unit dose (in individuals) or unit collective dose (in populations) of ionizing radiations have been evaluated especially by UNSCEAR and BEIR. Dose–response curves of genetic effects of both chemicals and radiations are at least approximately linear. It is therefore possible to use as a standard the risk associated with unit radiation dose in order to estimate risks of heritable damage and probably of cancer from exposure to chemicals. It will be shown that this risk evaluation in a purely submammalian system is possible under the following conditions:

1. The laboratory organism and man should exhibit the same similarities and differences in repair of initial damage from the agent under test and from ionizing radiation.

2. The organism should record forward mutation.

3. A reasonably correct assumption of the half-life of reactive compounds under test in human tissues, as a basis of a tissue dose estimate, is required.

4. If mammalian components, such as 'activating' liver enzymes, are not added to the system, the suggested risk estimate is only valid for primary mutagens/carcinogens, such as alkylating agents.

In tests of primarily non-reactive compounds which give rise to reactive products through chemical or metabolic conversion (demonstration of the latter requiring addition of metabolizing enzymes to the medium), risk estimates require knowledge of the dose – which may be defined as (duration of the treatment) × (average concentration during treatment) – both in the test organism and in man. The dose may be determined from the relative abundance of products of reaction with biological macromolecules.

It can be shown that the number of chemical changes per unit amount of DNA, which is associated with the same mutation frequency as is induced by unit dose of gamma-radiation, is the same in different organisms fulfilling condition (1) above, and the same for different monofunctional alkylating agents. This leads to the following two corollaries.

1. All chemicals which are alkylating, or which are converted *in vivo* to alkylating agents, are mutagenic and most probably carcinogenic.

2. At a given dose (defined above) the biological response is proportional to the rate of reaction with certain centres.

The resolving power of purely chemical tests is many orders of magnitude greater than that of biological test systems. Since, further, a determination of reaction products may be used directly, in conjunction with certain reaction kinetic data and certain correction factors (which have to be evaluated in forward-mutation systems), for a quantitation of risk, suitable chemical tests should be included in test batteries.

STATISTICAL ASPECTS ON TEST DATA AND QUANTITATION OF RISK

The development of test systems aims ultimately at providing better information on risks to man from environmental factors. A development of test systems is therefore required for effects not detected by systems already available, or if there are reasons to consider systems in use to be too insensitive, i.e. the probability of getting false negatives to be too high. What we need, above all, is test systems that permit us to quantitate the risk associated with given exposure levels of pollutants.

The three-tier system of Bridges[1] is a suitable frame for looking at these problems. If a compound has given positive results in one or a few of the genetic tests to which it has been subjected, if it is of considerable economical, technical or medical importance to man, and if there are no immediate substitutes for it, or no alternative known to be innocuous, administrators have to act in some way. (We assume that there is statistical and other evidence indicating that the probability of the positive tests being false is very small.) The following questions then arise.

Which possibilities do we have to draw conclusions from laboratory experiments as to the magnitude of risks to man (of cancer, heritable diseases or developmental damage) ?

This information is required for cost–benefit evaluations suggesting risks to be kept at a level that is reasonably low compared to the gain from using the compound, or for comparative cost–benefit analyses where risk associated with alternative solutions of a technical problem (such as, food preservation, energy generation) are compared[2].

Whereas positive tests mostly lead to some kind of action – and even a bad or incorrect action, which can be rectified later, is mostly better than no action at all – the interpretation of negative tests may turn out to be of greater concern: A great collective harm might originate from widespread pollutants with even a carcinogenic/mutagenic activity so weak that it remained undetected in laboratory tests.

This second problem is related to the fact that the dose–response of genetic effects is most correctly described in terms of a straight line with a finite slope already at dose zero. (In many cases dose–response curves appear to have a convex or concave shape; such deviations from linearity occur at relatively high doses, however, and a linear curve predominates at those low doses which are of primary interest in environmental health protection.) This means that there is no safe threshold dose below which mutation cannot be induced or cancer cannot be initiated. Also a negative test result, i.e. a difference $= 0$ between, say, mutation frequencies in a test sample and a control sample has an uncertainty which, in statistical terms, may be expressed by the confidence interval that covers the true value of the difference with a certain probability, often 95%. This confidence interval can be made smaller by increasing the size of a test, but it can never reach the value zero because of practical difficulties in increasing the number of test organisms beyond certain limits[3].

Any standardized biological test has therefore a characteristic 'resolving power', the inverse of the response that can be detected with a certain probability $(1-\beta)$ when, in the statistical evaluation of test data the hypothesis of no effect is rejected at a certain probability level $(a;$ often 5% or 1%)[3]. Against this background, the second question may be formulated.

Does a negative test exclude (at reasonably small probabilities a and β) a risk that would be non-acceptable to man?

Considering the linearity of dose–response curves and the uncertainty of negative tests, the classification of an environmental factor as 'non-mutagenic' ('non-carcinogenic', etc.) in contradistinction to mutagenic or

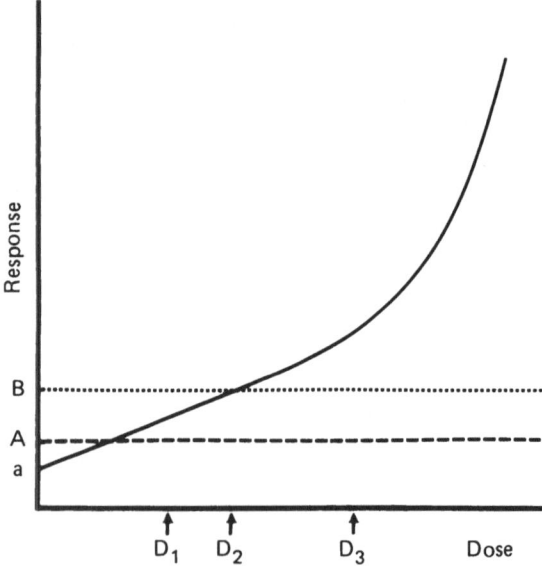

Figure 5.1 Illustration of a dose–response curve predominated at low doses by: Response $= a + b\,D$ ($a =$ spontaneous response). A = response corresponding to acceptable risk; B = response of the system detectable at reasonable values of a- and β-errors. The genetic toxicity of the compound in question will be detected at doses $>D_2$, e.g. D_3. If the highest dose that can be tested, e.g. because of acute toxicity, is D_1, the probability is great that the genetic toxicity remains undetected

carcinogenic requires additional information, beyond what is obtained from biological testing (see Figure 5.1). This conclusion is valid for all kinds of test systems. However, certain submammalian systems have the advantage that they can be manipulated towards higher sensitivity, and can, in critical cases, be run in an enlarged scale more easily than tests with mammals, thus minimizing the chances of erroneous conclusions from positive or negative tests.

USE OF RADIATION RISK AS A STANDARD

Radiation risk

The only environmental factor that has so far been evaluated with regard to risk coefficients for genetic effects, is ionizing radiation[4-6]. Considering dose–response curves to be linear (which is certainly approximately true at low-medium doses[5], these risk coefficients which have the dimension probability per man-rad*, may be used to estimate the risk (i.e. probability) that a person receiving a certain radiation dose will, in consequence of this exposures, develop a cancer or give rise to offspring with heritable disease. Also the expected number of cancer cases or cases of heritable diseases due to exposure of a population of size N to the average dose $\bar{D}$ may be computed. In this case the practical concept of collective dose ($N \times \bar{D}$ man-rad) is used. Likewise the exposure due to a certain activity such as a nuclear plant and the ensuing harm may be calculated (as the collective dose commitment and collective harm commitment, respectively)[7].

Dose of chemicals

To the extent that dose–response curves are linear, the same concepts would be applicable in cost–risk–benefit evaluations of other pollutants as well, including chemicals in the environment. It is then evident that the expected response, i.e. the risk, is related to dose (D) of a chemical which is the time (t) integral of concentration, $C(t)$[8,9]

$$D = \int_t C(t)\mathrm{d}t$$

(dimension: concentration $\times$ time)   (1)

*We retain here the old unit of radiation dose, rad (1 rad = 100 erg g^{-1}), because it is still generally used. In the SI system, unit radiation dose is 1 J kg^{-1} = 1 gray (Gy–; 1 Gy = 100 rad). Genetic risks are proportional to doses of γ- or X-radiation given in these units. More densely ionizing radiation (neutrons, α-rays) are mostly more effective, and doses are then multiplied by quality factors and become then expressed in the units 'rem' (roentgen-equivalent-man) and 'Sv' (sievert), respectively, which are proportional to risk[7].

Concentration is then an intensity parameter analogous to dose rate in exposure to ionizing radiation.

If a tested compound is so stable that the concentration may be considered constant during the period of treatment, the dose becomes simply the product of concentration and time (Figure 5.2).

$$D = C \times t \text{ mol l}^{-1}\text{h} \qquad (2)$$

Revell[10] demonstrated early that at equal doses $(C \times t)$ of diglycidyl ether, obtained at different concentrations C varied by a factor 60, the same frequency of chromosomal aberrations were induced in root tips of *Vicia faba*, and Kölmark and Kilbey[11] made the same observation for mutation induced by epoxides in *Neurospora* macrospores or microspores even at those high concentrations which give a non-linear dose–response.

For the evaluation of genetic risks of chemicals we are primarily

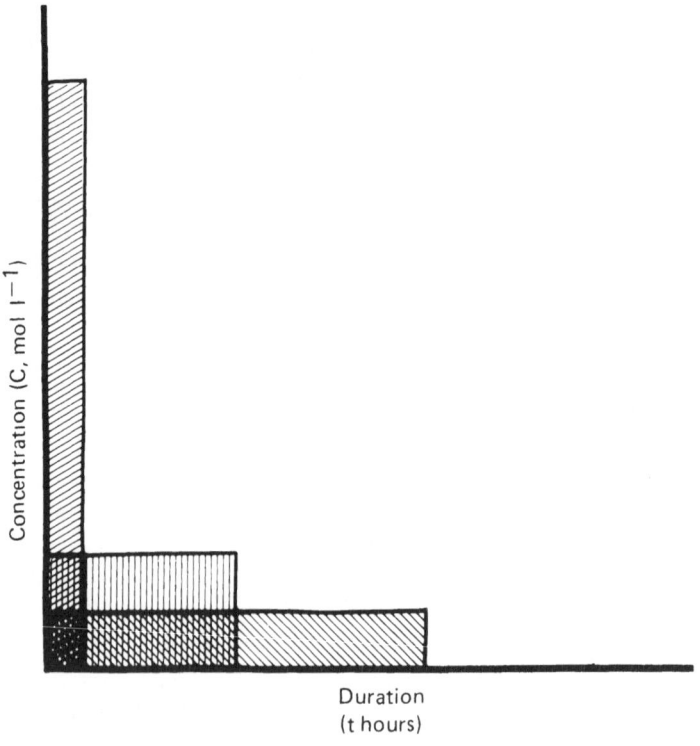

Duration
(t hours)

Figure 5.2　The same dose of a relatively stable compound applied at three different concentrations

interested in the dose of the proximal mutagen/carcinogen in target cells, or even in the nuclei of these cells (such as gonad cells in the case of heritable damage, or bone-marrow cells in the case of leukaemia). These doses, and their relationships to exposure doses may be measured directly in man from the degree of chemical change in macromolecules, e.g. haemoglobin, of known stability[12].

Figures 5.3 and 5.4 illustrate the distribution in time of dose following single injection into a mammal and in man respectively during a working week with intermittent exposure. In such cases the doses may be estimated from

$$D = \frac{C_0}{\lambda} \tag{3}$$

where C_0 is the hypothetical (total) absorbed or formed concentration (in mol $kg^{-1} \approx$ mol l^{-1}) of the proximal mutagen/carcinogen provided no elimination processes were in operation, and λ is the rate constant (in

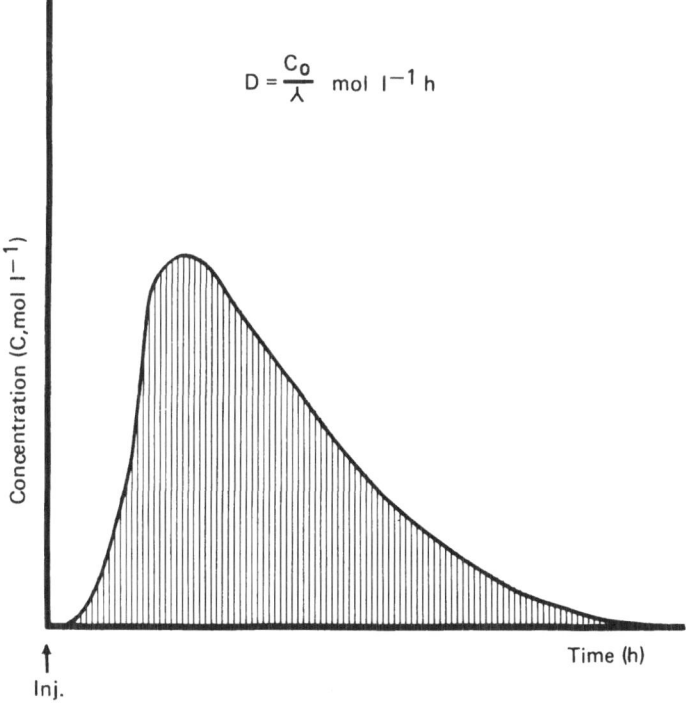

Figure 5.3 Illustration of the organ dose of a reactive metabolite formed from an injected compound. $C_0 =$ amount injected or amount converted to electrophile (in mol) divided by body weight (kg $\approx$ l).

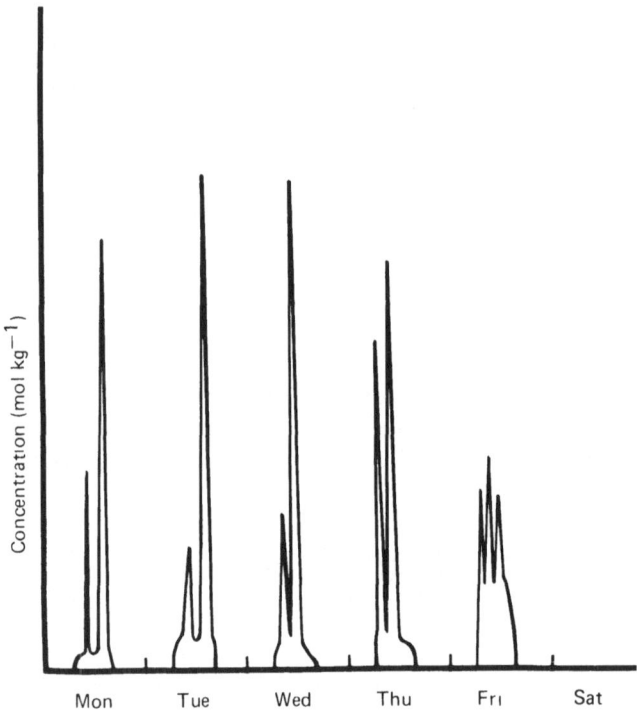

Figure 5.4 Illustration of the weekly dose, and its distribution in time, from a chemical giving the highest exposure concentration during a few daily operations of short duration (cf. [28]). The weekly dose may be calculated from:

$$D = \frac{\Sigma \text{ amount absorbed (mol)}}{\text{body weight (kg)}} \times \frac{1}{\lambda(\text{h}^{-1})} \text{ mol kg}^{-1}\text{h}$$

h^{-1}) of the processes of elimination from tissue approximated by a first-order reaction[8,12].

In certain cases a correction factor for 'unequal distribution in the body is required and has to be determined from animal experiments[13–14].

It is possible in only a few cases to determine risk coefficients for unit exposure dose of chemicals (for an air pollutant, e.g. 1 ppm h). For several reasons valuable information may at present be obtained from a use of risks associated with exposure to unit dose of γ-radiation (1 rad) as a standard expressing risks from exposure to chemicals[13]. Above all, ionizing radiation is a pollutant originating from natural as well as man-made sources, and permissible exposure levels (annual doses) in work-environments and to the public are based on the awareness of, and estimates of, genetic risks[7]. Expressing risks, from given doses of chemicals as well as the upper limits of risk in negative tests (cf. above), in rad-equivalents, will therefore give probability figures within a frame of reference to which administrators, politicians and the public are accustomed. It will further facilitate comparative risk estimates especially of nuclear and fossil energy, and give ideas on how to handle additive risks from radiations and other factors.

It is, however, clear that chemicals vary with regard to spectra of biological effects they produce, and that no chemical induces various biological effects in the same relative frequencies as are found in radiation experiments. The rad-equivalence, therefore, is rather a rough weapon which has to be used with caution. Several data indicate, on the other hand, that many of the 'specificities' of chemicals observed in experiments at high doses, are of limited practical interest, where, due to compound-specific acute toxicity, dose–response curves are no longer linear.

Resolving power of test systems

We can get an impression of the sensitivity of test systems by presenting the lowest radiation dose, the response of which we have a fair chance (1-β) to detect. In several test systems, run with standardized numbers of test organisms, the order of magnitude of this dose is 100 rad, if we reject the null-hypothesis at the 5% level (that is, allow the α-error, the probability of getting a false positive, to be as high as 1/20), and permitting the β-error to be in the range of 5–20%.

Particularly in cases where for some reason the agent cannot be tested with any safety margin, a negative test leaves us in the unsatisfactory position of knowing only that the agent with 80–95% probability is less dangerous than 100 rad of γ-radiation. This is the situation for example, with the possibly existing non-thermal effects of microwaves – because permissible levels are based on the ability of the body to get rid of heat. Another example is the higher alkenes (with 12–17 carbons), which occur in certain foods and are formed from lipids when foods are preserved by irradiation[15]. Because of a low solubility, a slow rate of penetration into cells, a low dose of the epoxides which are the electrophilic metabolites, and a low reactivity of the epoxide groups, it is hardly possible in a standard test to detect the mutagenic action of these compounds. A third example is dichlorvos, demonstrated in micro-organisms to be mutagenic, but which, because of the toxicity in consequence of cholinesterase inhibition, can be subjected to cancer test only at doses so low that no tumour induction can be expected anyway.

In these and similar cases evidence from other sources is required for a quantitative evaluation of the genetic toxicity, and particularly in the microwave case, to establish whether such a toxicity at all exists.

Reaction-kinetic model

Alkylating and other electrophilic reagents react at random with nucleophilic groups in the cells, but in a dependence on the nucleophilic strength of these groups which may be described by the Swain–Scott model[16–18]. This empirical free energy relationship related reaction rate k_n at nucleophilicity n to the rate of reaction with water through

$$\log k_n = \log k_{H_2O} + s \cdot n \qquad (4)$$

where the substrate constant, s, of methyl bromide was set $= 1$. Of important nucleophiles in tissue, sulphurs $(-S^-)$ have n-values in the range 5–7, nitrogens $(-NR_2)$ in the range 3–6, oxygens (-0^-) in the range 1–4, and n of chloride (Cl^-) is 3.0 (cf.[16] and quoted literature). S-values are high (>1) for 'sulphydryl inhibitors' such as iodoacetamide, low for S_N1-type reactants (such as isopropyl methanesulphonate and the reactive principles from nitrosamides and nitrosamines), and have intermediate values (0.6–1.0) for the majority of standard mutagens (ethylene oxide 0.96; methyl methanesulphonate 0.89; ethyl methanesulphonate 0.69[16]). For a number of relatively simple, monofunctional alkylating agents the mutagenic effectiveness (i.e. slopes of dose–response curves in the linear regions) or mutation frequency per unit dose, D, was found to be proportional to the rate of reaction, $k_{n=2}$, at a relatively low nucleophilicity, $n \approx 2$. This value may represent a mean of some groups in DNA, including guanine-O^6, of a relatively low reactivity compared to that of the most reactive centre, guanine-N-7 $(n = 3.5)$.

Considering a general nucleophilic substitution reaction:

$$RX + Y^- \rightarrow RY + Y^- \qquad (5)$$

proceeding with rate k, the product $D \times k$ is in fact equal to the degree of alkylation, $[RY]/[Y^-]$, of the nucleophilic centre, Y^-. One may then ask which degree of alkylation of the hypothetical low-reactivity centres, $Y_{n=2}$, is associated with the same mutation frequency as is obtained with

1 rad of γ-radiation. Within a factor 2, for the simple agents discussed, this degree of alkylation is found to be one in ten million, i.e.

$$1 \text{ rad} \leftrightarrow \frac{[RY_{n=2}]}{[Y_{n=2}^-]} = D \times k_{n=2} = 1 \cdot 10^{-7} \tag{6}$$

This relationship is evidently approximately valid for bacteria such as *Escherichia coli* and, according to work with ethyl methanesulphonate, *Mycobacterium phlei*[20], higher plants (barley) as well as mammals.

When computing risk, correction has to be done for functionality (difunctional or polyfunctional agents being one to two orders of magnitude more effective per initial alkylation[21]); steric effects (not the least, consequences of intercalation), lipid–water partition coefficients[19], distribution in body, etc.[13]. Collecting these correction factors, f_i, as a product ($\prod_i$), a general risk expression may be formulated

$$\text{risk} = D \times k_{n=2} \times 1 \cdot 10^7 \times \prod_i f_i \text{ rad equ.} \tag{7}$$

For certain simple monofunctional agents such as ethylene oxide and methyl methanesulphonate the product $\prod_i f_i$ may be set equal to one.

The rad-equivalence of submammalian systems: validity to man?

Comparing the slopes of the linear regions of dose–response curves in *Escherichia coli* Sd-4 and in germinating barley karyopses obtained in experiments with γ-radiation (or X-rays) and with alkylating agents, the rad-equivalence, the radiation dose that gives the same response as unit chemical dose (for practical reasons often given in mM $\times$ h, i.e. mmol $\times$ 1^{-1} $\times$ h), attains approximately the same value in the two systems, for example

Methyl methanesulphonate: 6×10^2 rad (mM $\times$ h)
Ethylene oxide: 1.2×10^2 rad (mM $\times$ h)

For these two chemicals the tissue dose in the mouse, per unit absorbed dose, was determined by means of the degree of alkylation of haemoglobin and verified by the degree of alkylation of DNA. The doses of these compounds, per unit absorbed chemical (expressed as 'initial concentration', C_0) correspond to rates of elimination, λ, and biological half-lives, $t_{\frac{1}{2}}$, according to:

	λ	$t_{\frac{1}{2}}$	D* per mmol $\times$ kg^{-1} $\times$ mM(h)
Methyl methanesulphonate	1.3–2.0 h^{-1}	20–30 min	0.5–0.7
Ethylene oxide	4.6 h^{-1}	9 min	0.22

For a number of endpoints obtained following experimental exposure of mice and/or rats to these two chemicals, practically the same rad-equivalence was computed, as in the above-mentioned experiments with *Escherichia coli* and barley. These endpoints comprise chromosomal aberrations in various organs and dominant-lethal mutations[21], and the frequency of specific locus mutations induced by methyl methanesulphonate does not disagree with this ratio[16]. Assuming that a few derivatives of ethylene oxide have the same value of λ as the unsubstituted compound, further support was obtained for the idea that the rad-equivalence has the same value in submammalian and mammalian systems. Therefore, it may be assumed that values of rad-equivalence thus established could be applied, at least as a first approximation, in estimates of risk of heritable damage in man.

Too few data are at hand to decide whether the same values of the rad-equivalence are valid for initiation of cancer, but preliminary data from experiments with methylating agents and epoxides in animal strains judged to be related to those used in the radiation experiments indicate that this is the case[13,21]. The cancer incidence in a group of persons exposed occupationally to ethylene oxide was predicted on the basis of tissue doses monitored by haemoglobin alkylation and applying the risk coefficient for leukaemia induction by radiation, and seems to have been confirmed epidemiologically[21,22]. This would be expected if the mutation theory of cancer initiation is valid.

Values for the rad-equivalence would be valid generally if ABCW-type curves[23], that is, linear dependences on the amount of DNA per genome, of the mutation frequency per locus, are obtained with chemicals as well as with radiation[24]. Deviating values would further be obtained for systems such as *Micrococcus radiodurans* and *Schizosaccharomyees pombe* which have an 'abnormal' ability to repair radiation damage[13].

Electrophilic reactivity as a criterion of genetic toxicity

The demonstration above that

$$\text{mutation frequency} \propto D \times k_{n=2} \qquad (8)$$

*$D = C_0/\lambda$; for original data, see [8,29].

leads to the important corollary that any compound that is, or can be, converted by metabolism or chemical reaction to an alkylating agent is mutagenic, and most likely also carcinogenic. Probably, this concerns other types of electrophilic reactivity as well (for example, acylation, Schiff-base formation by aldehydes).

The resolving power of the demonstration, *in vivo* or *in vitro*, of products of nucleophilic substitution is many orders of magnitude higher than that of any biological test[25]. In particular, a high sensitivity is obtained when work can be carried out with radioactively labelled compounds, permitting the detection of responses corresponding to less than 1 millirad-equivalent, thus eliminating the uncertainty and uneasiness of certain negative biological tests. It is therefore suggested that suitable chemical systems are introduced in the evaluation of genetic risks from environmental chemicals. One advantage of such chemical tests is that they may be immediately useful for quantitative risk estimates.

If a confirmation on the biological level is wanted, the expected frequency of genetic events in a given exposure situation may be computed, and the scope of a test required for the detection of this response estimated[3]. The computed expected frequency can further be applied as the contrahypothesis in estimating the β-error of negative tests. It was shown through an approach of this kind that negative tests of some epoxides for the ability to induce dominant-lethal mutations or tumours, did not prove that the compounds were non-mutagenic or non-carcinogenic and the tests were less effective than expected from reaction kinetic data[21].

DATA REQUIRED FOR RISK ESTIMATES

Since genetic risks depend on doses in human target organs certain information from mammalian systems is obligatory for risk estimates. This information pertains, however, to the kind and amount of proximal mutagen/carcinogen rather than to observed biological endpoints. If we therefore define a system as submammalian on the basis of the endpoint used to measure biological effectiveness (as in the cases of micro-organisms tested in the presence of tissue extract, or tested in a host-mediated assay), such systems combined with information on the relationship of human tissue doses to exposure dose or uptake, would permit risk estimates which are, at least, better than nothing.

Primary mutagens/carcinogens, especially alkylating agents, present in risk estimates a somewhat simpler case than secondary agents rendered reactive through metabolic conversion. To the extent that assumptions as to the rate of elimination – λ of equation (3) – and distribution in the body can be made on the basis of experience from related compounds[21], a risk estimate could be based on a forward mutation test with micro-organisms, carried out under conditions permitting control of concentration during the treatment – for example, liquid suspension preferable to plate test. Knowing the response of the system to γ-radiation, a dose-response curve obtained in a positive test may then be recalculated directly to rad-equivalence, including chemical and biochemical correction factors (i.a., for steric effects and functionality). For compounds of such low reactivity that tests become negative, risks will have to be estimated solely from reaction-kinetic parameters (and dose parameters), and values of correction factors have then to be based on experience from work with compounds of related structure.

The main importance of biological tests lies in the evaluation of correction factors. In this field, much more research is required; for instance, it is not clear to what extent isolated DNA or bacterial DNA correctly reflects the reactivity of the DNA of mammalian nucleoproteins[19].

In the case of chemicals which are non-reactive *per se* but which give rise to mutagenic/carcinogenic metabolites, doses of the proximal mutagens/carcinogens are strongly dependent on the organization and induction status of activating and deactivating enzymes. It cannot be expected, therefore, that any experimental system, be it micro-organisms tested in the presence of mammalian enzymes or even intact mammals[26] will serve as a sufficiently accurate model of man. Methods should therefore be developed to determine doses directly in man, for example, from the degree of alkylation or other chemical change in haemoglobin or, if possible, sperm DNA[12]. If the reactive metabolites are known, as, for instance, in the case of epoxides formed from 1-alkenes[27], risk estimates could be based on biological and/or chemical tests of these compounds. If they are unknown, they might be identified from reaction products with rodent or human haemoglobin *in vivo* or with proteins of bacteria tested in the presence of mammalian enzymes. If the compound is not available with radioactive label – this is always the case with complex samples of air pollution, extracts from foods, etc. – incorporation of labelled histidine into proteins (a completely specific incorporation into *Salmonella typhimurium his⁻* bacteria is possible), or labelled guanine into DNA offers a suitable system for the demonstration of genetic toxicity and, if this toxicity is sufficiently great, for the establishment of dose–response curves by the measurement of reaction products with labelled component and of mutation frequency in the same experiment. Until more is known about similarities and differences between man and laboratory animals with regard to metabolizing enzymes, such dose–response curves should preferably be established with representative human enzyme preparations, at least as a complement to preparations from laboratory animals.

References

 1. Bridges, B. A. (1973). Some general principles of mutagenicity screening and a possible framework for testing procedures, *Environ. Hlth Perspect.*, **6**, 221
 2. Ehrenberg, L. (1974). Genetic toxicity of environmental chemicals, *Acta Biol. Iugosl. Ser. F Genetika*, **6**, 367
 3. Ehrenberg, L. (1977). Aspects of statistical inference in testing for genetic toxicity, In B. Kilbey *et al.* (eds.). *Handbook of Mutagenicity Test Procedures*, pp. 420–458. (Amsterdam: Elsevier/North Holland)
 4. BEIR. (1972). The effects on populations of exposure to low levels of ionizing radiation, (Washington: National Academy of Sciences)
 5. Ehrenberg, L. (1978). Dose–response relationship for biological effects of ionizing radiation: Application in risk estimation (Dos–respons samband för biologiska effekter av joniserande strålning : tillämpning vid riskupp-skattning), (Stockholm: Report to the Swedish Energy Commission)
 6. UNSCEAR, United Nations Scientific Committee on the Effects of Atomic Radiation. (1977). *Sources and Effects of Ionizing Radiation*, (New York: United Nations)
 7. ICRP. (1977). *Recommendations of the International Commission on Radiological Protection, Publ.* **26**, (Oxford: Pergamon Press)
 8. Ehrenberg, L., Hiesche, K. D., Osterman-Golkar, S. and Wennberg, I. (1974). Evaluation of genetic risks of alkylating agents: Tissue dose in the mouse from air contaminated with ethylene oxide, *Mutat. Res.*, **24**, 83
 9. Latarjet, R. (1977). Quantitative mutagenesis by chemicals and by radiations: Prerequisites for the establishment of rad-equivalences, In R. Chanet (ed.) *Radiological Protection, First Eur. Symp. on Rad-Equivalence*, pp. 154–168. (Luxembourg: Commission of the European Communities)
10. Revell, S. H., Chromosome breakage by X-rays and radiomimetic substances in *Vicia. Heredity*, Suppl. 6 (1953) 107
11. Kölmark, H. G. and Kilbey, B. J. (1968). Kinetic studies of mutation induction, by epoxides in *Neurospora crassa, Molec. Gen. Genet.*, **101**, 89
12. Osterman-Golkar, S., Ehrenberg, L. Segerbäck, D. and Hällström, (1976). Evaluation of genetic risks of alkylating agents. II. Haemoglobin as a dose monitor, *Mutat. Res.*, **34**, 1
13a. Ehrenberg, L. (1978). Methods of comparing risks of radiation and chemicals: the rad-equivalence of stochastic effects of chemicals. (Vienna: IAEA) (In press)
13b. Ehrenberg, L. (1978). Purposes and methods of comparing effects of radiation and chemicals. (Vienna: IAEA) (In press)
14. Hussain, S. and Ehrenberg, L. (1977). Gene mutations: Dose–response relationships and their significance for extrapolation to man, *Abh. Akad. Wiss. DDR*, No. N9, 95
15. Chinn, H. I. (1977), Committee Chairman. Evaluation of the health aspects of certain compounds found in irradiated beef. (Bethesda, Maryland: Life

88 MUTAGENESIS IN SUB-MAMMALIAN SYSTEMS

Sciences Research Office, Federation of American Societies for Experimental Biology)
16. Osterman-Golkar, S. (1975). Studies on the reaction kinetics of biologically active electrophilic reagents as a basis for risk estimates, Thesis, Stockholm University
17. Osterman-Golkar, S., Ehrenberg, L. and Wachtmeister, C. A. (1970). Reaction kinetics and biological action in barley of monofunctional methanesulfonic esters, *Radiation Bot.*, **10**, 303
18. Swain, C. G. and Scott, C. B. (1953). Quantitative correlation of relative rates. Comparison of hydroxide ion with other nucleophilic reagents toward alkyl halides, esters, epoxides and acyl halides. *J. Am. Chem. Soc.*, **75**, 141
19. Djalali-Behzad, Gh., *et al.* (1979) Genetic risk of methyl bromide. (In preparation)
20. Kolman, A. and Ehrenberg, L. (1978). Induction of a morphological mutant in *Mycobacterium phlei* by gamma-radiation and ethyl methanesulfonate, *Mutat. Res.*, **49**, 297
21. Ehrenberg, L., and Hussain, H. (1979). Genetic toxicity of some important epoxides. (Submitted)
22. Calleman, C. J., Ehrenberg, L., Jansson, B., Osterman-Golkar, S. Segerbäck, D., Svensson, K. and Wachtmeister, C. A. (1978). Monitoring and risk assessment by means of haemoglobin alkylation in persons occupationally exposed to ethylene oxide, *J. Toxicol. Environ. Hlth* (In press)
23. Abrahamson, S., Bender, M. A., Conger, A. D. and Wolff, S. (1973). Uniformity of radiation-induced mutation rates among different species. *Nature (London)*, **245**, 460
24. Heddle, J. A. (1978). Extrapolation of mutation rate data from experimental organisms to man. (Vienna: IAEA) (In press)
25. Ehrenberg, L. and Osterman-Golkar, S. (1977). Reaction kinetics of chemical pollutants as a basis of risk estimates in terms of rad-equivalents, In R. Chanet (ed.) *Radiological Protection, First Eur. Symp. on Rad-Equivalence*, pp. 199–205 (Luxembourg: Commission of the European Communities)
26. Ehrenberg, L. and Holmberg, B. (1978). Extrapolation of carcinogenic risk from animal experiments to man, *Environ. Hlth Perspectives*, **22**, 33
27. Ehrenberg, L., Osterman-Golkar, S., Segerbäck, D. Svensson, K., and Calleman, C. J. Evalution of the genetic risks of alkylating agents. III. Alkylation of haemoglobin after metabolic conversion of ethene to ethene oxide *in vivo*, *Mutat. Res.*, **45**, 175
28. Dunkelberg, H. and Hartmetz, G. (1977). Zur Belastung der Raumluft durch Äthylenoxid im Bereich klinischer Sterilisationsanlagen (Recording the air pollution by ethylene oxide in clinical sterilization installations), *Zbl. Bakt. Hyg., I. Abt. Orig. B* **164**, 271
29. Segerbäck, D., Calleman, C. J., Ehrenberg, L., Löfroth, G., and Osterman-Golkar, S., Evaluation of genetic risks of alkylating agents. IV. Quantitative determination of alkylated amino acids in haemoglobin as a measure of the dose after treatment of mice with methyl methanesulfonate, *Mutat. Res.*, **49**, (1978) 71

Discussion
Chairman: Professor B. A. Bridges

Professor D. V. PARKE (Guildford): On the last matter mentioned by Professor Ehrenberg about the rates of metabolic activation of secondary carcinogens and mutagens, this is of paramount importance. Professor Ehrenberg has put his finger on the most important aspect since there is accumulating evidence that the rates of microsomal oxidative metabolism activation of these carcinogens and mutagens in small rodents like mice and rats is very much faster, 10 or 20 times faster, than in man and primates, and the epoxide hydrase which will deactivate these is very much lower. So we shall get considerable magnification of the hazard when we use rats and mice as models for man, and I should like to see more work done in the primates.

In the US, Dick Andersen has shown that he can testing reasonably strong carcinogens get a response in half a dozen primate species within 2 years. It is therefore quite needless to consider lifespan studies for carcinogenicity testing where we are only looking for the really important carcinogens.

On that same aspect, when Professor Ames mentioned epidemiology, as Professor Ehrenberg said, it is a matter of dose, and exposure, rather than some arbitrary value of how long it will take before the carcinogens are developed. It is well known in animals, it has been publicized for 30 or

40 years, but it is strange how many people think that man will not manifest malignancy till some 25 years after exposure. I know that Professor Ames does not agree with this.

The recent work which has been published in the US on cyclophosphamide and various other alkylating agents which are used in the treatment of malignant disease in man has shown leukaemia – myeloid leukaemia particularly – coming up in 5 years.

Professor BRIDGES: But those are massive doses – those cytostatic drug data in humans. The one thing that we know is that the latent period decreases as the dose is increased. Since in the environment the doses are likely to be more modest, one would expect longer latent periods.

Professor D. V. PARKE: I appreciate that. I am not contradicting that at all. What I am saying is that there are many clinicians – most of my colleagues, I regret to say, on the CSM – who have held the point of view that a medicine which was known to be a mutagen, an alkylating agent, possibly would not produce any dire results in man in perhaps 20–25 years.

Professor BRIDGES: I would agree with you there, because medicines are given at very significant doses.

Professor PARKE: What worries me is that many of these alkylating agents are prescribed as medicines for psoriasis and skin conditions. We have agreed to their use for serious skin conditions, but these very powerful mutagens and carcinogens are being used by some physicians for much less serious conditions.

Professor L. EHRENBERG (Stockholm): To comment on dose levels. It is rather remarkable to find in workers in an ethylene oxide sterilization plant such amounts of chemically changed haemoglobin that has reacted with the ethylene oxide to give rise to hydroxyethylhistidine as one amino acid – and in such an amount that it could be determined by an amino acid analyser without any necessity to go to a mass spectrometer or some more sophisticated method so as to determine it.

I wrote exposure to 1 ppm for 1 hour corresponds to 10 mrad in effect. The maximum permissible weekly dose for radiological workers in most western countries is 100 mrad. The maximum permissible weekly dose for an ethylene oxide worker who works at top level is around 20 rad equivalents in most countries, or about 200 times the risk run by the radiological worker. Those workers in whom we measured chemically changed haemoglobin worked at about one-third of the traditional level. For many chemicals in the work environment, the exposure dose levels or the exposure concentrations are so high that the risk could be measured directly by measuring changes in the haemoglobin long before the cancer develops. Any compound which gives rise to an alkylating amino acid is certainly a mutagen, and most probably also a carcinogen.

There are analytical methods sufficiently sensitive to measure reactions for a great number of chemicals in urban areas which are just general pollutants in these areas, and I am quite positive about the possibilities of known pollutants having dose levels which are of interest to the public generally.

Professor Ivo de CARNERI (Milan): Is having a choice of studies, such as *E. coli*, yeast methods, etc. of any help?

Professor B. N. AMES (Berkeley): It is worth having a battery of tests. It may be that one wants mammalian cell tests in addition to *Salmonella* plus one method demonstrating chromosomol damage. People are now discussing which group of these would make the best group of tests.

Professor BRIDGES: One point on which it is worth spending some time is the question of the response of man to a given mutagenic challenge. We do not know. For example, with Professor Ehrenberg's approach in ethylene oxide and these other epoxides, measurements of rad equivalence can be made, and this is worth doing. There is no doubt about that.

But, one cannot assume that the effect of 1 rad equivalent of ethylene oxide will be the same in man as 1 rad of radiation, because they are very different in their consequences in DNA. It seems to me that one of the things that we must start doing is to calibrate the human response. We must start to tie in our epidemiology with our life studies. It is really quite a new idea, and one that has to come. We are now beginning to see the techniques in the laboratory where we can do it.

Professor Ehrenberg's technique of looking at alkylations of histidine in haemoglobin is one of the early markers. It occurs right after exposure, and it persists for a long time, and it can be measured. The exposure of people can be measured. That is something that can be tied in with epidemiology. Biological responses in man can also be tied in. I mentioned cytogenetics and I mentioned the new technique (Albertini and Strauss) for looking at gene mutations in peripheral lymphocytes. It is interesting, in view of what Professor Parkes said, that Albertini and Strauss looked at patients with psoriasis who had been treated with chemical mutagens as part of their treatment, and the level of HGPRT mutants in their lymphocytes was elevated at least ten-fold over the control population. So here again one could identify populations who were being treated and had been treated with mutagens, and one could escalate their doses, not only bio-chemically, or chemically, with histidine alkylation, but also biologically, by looking at the responses of their somatic cells. When we can tie that in, in just a few examples, with some epidemiological data, which nobody really has made any attempt to look for seriously, then we can begin to calibrate man and begin to put figures on the risks. But at the moment we are talking about a black box – Professor Ehrenberg may not agree.

Professor EHRENBERG: I partly agree with Professor Bridges. Because of shortage of time I could not dwell on these topics. Professor Bridges said that we could not expect 1 rad of radiation in man to give the same response as 1 rad equivalence of ethylene oxide. The rad equivalence we used was based on forward mutation tests in *E. coli*. If we used this rad equivalence and radiation data for dominant lethal mutations and chromo-some aberrations in the mouse and the rat, and for specific locus mutations in the mouse, we got exactly the predicted frequencies. If we used this dosage regime, taking into consideration the length of life of the chemical in the body – not milligrams injected or something similar, because that depends to such a high degree on the metabolism of the chemical – then if we knew what 1 rad of radiation would cause per million persons in man, we could predict the effect of a dose of the chemical in a like population.

SECTION THREE

Other Mutagenesis Test Systems

6

Sub-mammalian tests other than the Ames test for mutagenesis
Diana Anderson

INTRODUCTION

The possibility that genetic damage or mutations may be induced after exposure to chemicals is worrying not only to the scientist but also to the population at large.

Each year many different new chemicals are introduced into man's environment due to technical and scientific progress and some of these may be capable of inducing mutations. Mutations are stable and heritable modifications of the genetic information. Those occurring in somatic cells are only transmissible at the cellular level while those occurring in reproductive cells may be transmitted to successive generations. Thus with the revived interest in the somatic mutation theory of cancer and since many mutagens have been shown to be carcinogens[1–8], the study of the genetic effect of chemical substances may be useful not only for protecting the genetic integrity of future generations but also for preventing unnecessary exposure to potential carcinogens in the present generation.

Whilst cancer in man is an emotive issue and has a demonstrable link with chemical exposure, no such link has been unequivocally established for heritable genetic damage in man.

It is difficult, therefore, to determine the human significance of chemical mutagenicity results *in vitro*. However, it has been estimated that there is a genetic element in at least 10% of all human pathological conditions[9] so that genetic changes, if produced in man, could be serious.

Genetic abnormalities arise as a result of gene or chromosome mutation. Carter has described the relative contribution of mutant genes and chromosome abnormalities to genetic ill-health in man[10]. McKusick[11] has segregated 'traits' inherited at the level of the gene as dominant or recessive autosomal or sex-linked, dependent upon whether the mutant genes are located on autosomal or sex-linked chromosomes. Whilst the appearance of a dominant mutant gene is immediately expressed in the next generation (for example Huntington's chorea and achondroplasia), recessive mutations may take many generations to be expressed (such as phenylketonuria), except sex-linked recessives such as haemophilia. Many constitutional and degenerative diseases like epilepsy or schizophrenia may be caused by irregularities of gene expression or arise from multiple genes.

Chromosome abnormalities may arise either by errors in the distribution of chromosomes leading to abnormalities of chromosome numbers such as non-disjunction (Down's syndrome (mongolism), Klinefelter's and Turners's syndrome), for example where the effect is seen in the next generation or by the consequence of chromosome breakage (such as ataxia telangiectasia and Fanconi's anaemia). Some chromosome mutations are thought to give rise to early embryonic loss and they have little impact on society. Deleterious mutations which are capable of survival may be a heavy burden to society if the affected person requires medical or institutional care (mongolism, for example, which occurs in 1 in 1000 births in man). The different types of genetic damage and examples of the diseases which might arise are shown in Figure 6.1.

Thus, although it is not possible at present to give a quantitative estimate of the contribution of chemical agents to the incidence of genetic disease, it is probable that they are or could become an aetiological factor in such disease, and that the exposure of the human population to a growing number of possible mutagens must be viewed with concern. Hence, there is a need to define by means of appropriate tests the mutagenic activity of chemical substances as a part of their general toxicological evaluation. It must be remembered, however, that the evaluation of mutagenic effects is a complex and extremely difficult task and that no single method gives conclusive information about the genetic risk to a person who has been exposed to a mutagenic substance. Various recommendations for combinations of test systems have been put forward[12-26] and various governmental agencies such as those in Britain, Holland, Italy and other EEC

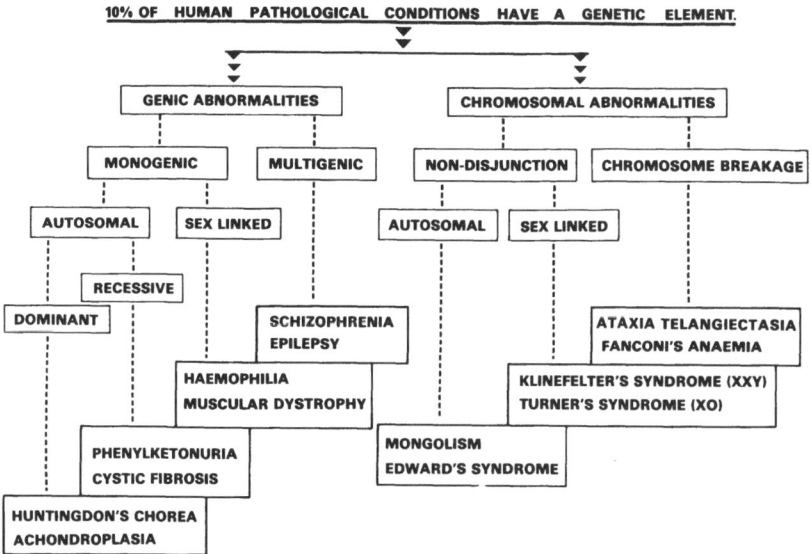

Figure 6.1   Examples of genetically based human pathological conditions

countries, America, Canada and Japan, are now preparing guidelines for testing methods.

Genetic material – deoxyribonucleic acid (DNA) – which is the critical target of mutagenic action, is substantially identical at the molecular level in all living organisms and this partially justifies the use of any organism in experimental studies; therefore various testing methods employ a large variety of organisms. However, there are differences in the organization of the genetic material in cells, on the basis of which some organisms may be considered more similar to man than others and thus more suitable for the purpose of evaluating human genetic risk. The existence in man of many factors which affect the mutagenic efficiency of a compound (concentration, absorption, distribution, stability, transport, penetration and metabolism in the target cell, reaction with DNA, immunological or repair mechanisms, detoxification and excretion in the organism, etc.) make it very difficult to extrapolate to man effects observed in experimental organisms or biological systems. Nevertheless, such data do indicate the mutagenic/carcinogenic *potential* of a compound.

The main sub-mammalian test systems currently available are briefly described and discussed below. These must be considered as those which reflect the present-day state of knowledge and they may therefore be improved with the progress of experimental work in this specific field. Not all of the available tests are described but a selection of them will be considered according to three categories, namely: (1) tests for gene mutation, (2) tests for chromosome damage, and (3) tests for DNA repair.

TESTS FOR GENE MUTATION

Gene mutations are defined as heritable alterations to the DNA. In molecular terms they consist of the substitution, deletion or insertion of one or more nucleotide base-pairs in the DNA. Mutations due to substitution are known as base-pair substitutions and those due to deletions or insertions as frameshifts. When a base-pair substitution mutation occurs a wrong base is inserted which then pairs with its natural partner during replication (adenine with thymine, cytosine with guanine) so that a new pair of incorrect bases is inserted in the DNA. When a frameshift mutation occurs, due to base-pair loss, then the DNA, which is read in triplet codons, incorporates the first base-pair from the next triplet codon (Figure 6.2). Thus

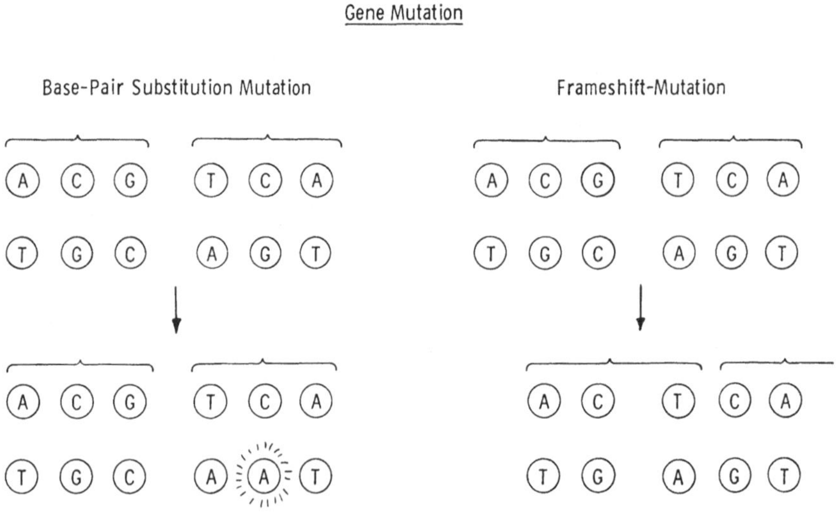

Gene Mutation

Base-Pair Substitution Mutation   Frameshift-Mutation

Figure 6.2 Mechanisms of gene mutation

the subsequent code of the DNA becomes scrambled until a nonsense or terminating codon is reached. Gene or point mutations cannot be detected by cytological methods but can be distinguished as variants of characteristics controlled by specific gene loci or as recessive lethal conditions (generally linked to the sex chromosome). Mutations of specific sites can

Gene Mutation

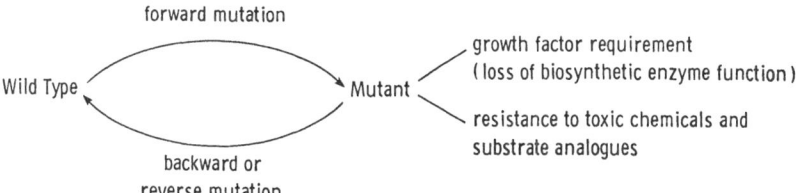

Figure 6.3   Detection of gene mutation

arise in either a 'backward' (from mutant to wild type) or a 'forward' direction (from wild type to mutant) (Figure 6.3).

Backward (reverse) mutation is generally studied in mutant cells which have known base-pair substitutions or frameshift mutations. Normal functional activity is re-established following a new substitution or a second deletion and insertion near the first one. Backward mutation is highly specific in the type of DNA interaction required and a chemical compound which does not increase the frequency of this type of mutation may nevertheless still cause other genetic effects.

Forward mutation may arise from substitutions, insertions, or deletions of the nucleotide bases of a gene, to deletion of the entire gene and neighbouring genes. They are detected when there is a loss of an enzyme function required for biosynthesis resulting in a growth factor requirement (auxotrophy) or from resistance to various toxic chemicals, substrate analogues and agents such as heat. In some cases, for example, with some genes controlling resistance, where only one specific locus may be affected, the forward mutation system can be just as restrictive as the backward mutation system in the sense that only very specific molecular changes can be detected.

The specificity of some of these mutation systems, together with secondary factors such as the effect of the particular nucleotide sequence near the original mutation makes a quantitative comparison or extrapolation of the mutagenicity of different chemicals very difficult. For a list of other factors which can influence mutagenic effects *in vitro* see Ashby and Styles (1978)[27].

Tests in micro-organisms

Tests in bacteria

Point mutations can be detected in various bacterial species. Those most commonly used are *Salmonella typhimurium, Escherichia coli* and *Streptomyces coelicolor*.

As well as its use in the reverse mutation assay of Ames detecting histidine independence, *Salmonella typhimurium* can be used for detecting forward mutations to 8-azaguanine resistance[28] and arabinose resistance[29]. *Escherichia coli* can be used for

1. The induction of base mutations from arginine dependence to independence[30] (base-pair substitution reverse mutation) or from tryptophan dependence to independence[31] (frame-shift reverse mutation).

2. The induction of forward mutations from inability to ability to ferment galactose[32] and from sensitivity to resistance to 5-methyltryptophan[33] or streptomycin[34]. These forward systems allow the detection of base-pair substitutions, frameshift mutations or small deletions.

3. The induction of prophage (inductest) which induces the stimulation of the lytic cycle in bacterial cells harbouring a latent bacteriophage so bringing about alterations which lead to destruction or deactivation of the phage repressor. These effects can be observed in a single strain which carries the necessary genetic markers and the bacteriophage in a prophage form[35]. However, it has been concluded that the inductest is not a very promising procedure for routine use in detecting environmental agents since only three out of 20 chemicals responded positively in this test whereas all were detected by the *Salmonella* assay[36].

4. Detecting mutation by means of a fluctuation test[37] which measures reverse mutation to tryptophan independence where only tryptophan revertants grow and cause turbidity in tubes and non-revertant tubes remain clear.

Streptomyces coelicolor can be used for the induction of forward mutations from streptomycin sensitivity to resistance[38].

Tests in fungi

The yeasts *Saccharomyces cerevisiae* and *Schizosaccharomyces pombe* and the Ascomycetes *Neurospora crassa* and *Aspergillus nidulans* are among the fungi most used for the detection of point mutations.

In the yeasts *Saccharomyces cerevisiae* and *Schizosaccharomyces pombe* mutations at each of the two genetic loci which control adenine biosynthesis cause a red pigmentation of the colonies. In *Saccharomyces cerevisiae* the effect has been used to develop forward mutation tests either in haploid or diploid strains. In the latter system as well as genetic analysis it is possible to distinguish the effect of the mutation from that of mitotic recombination by established morphological criteria. *Schizosaccharomyces pombe* has been used to detect forward mutation in wild or adenine-dependent haploid strains where mutations can be assessed in five genes simultaneously. Further mutations have been introduced into this strain which increase sensitivity to chemical mutagens. The use of these two yeasts for mutagenicity assays has been extensively reviewed[39–42]. A system of forward mutation from sensitivity to canavanine resistance[43] has also been developed in *Saccharomyces cerevisiae*. Cultures of *Saccharomyces cerevisiae* can also be used in a fluctuation test[44], for example, the D-7 strain is used for from isoleucine dependence to independence.

Strains of *Neurospora crassa* can be used for the induction of forward mutation in each of two genetic loci which control adenine biosynthesis[45] in a similar way to that described for yeasts. However, in addition strains have been developed which allow identification of (1) recessive point mutations at each of the two genetic loci mentioned; (2) dominant lethal mutations in the genetic region in which the two loci are situated; and (3) recessive mutations in the whole genome. The use of *Neurospora* for mutagenicity testing has been reviewed[45–47].

Strains of *Aspergillus nidulans* can be used for the induction of (1) forward mutation to 8-azaguanine and *p*-fluorophenlyalanine and (2) back mutation from methionine dependence to independence[48].

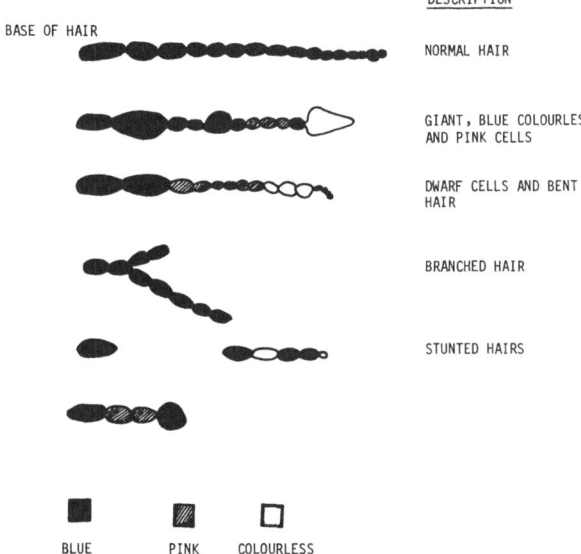

Figure 6.4 Diagram of a normal *Tradescantia* stamen hair and examples of aberrant hair and cell types following mutagen treatment

Tests in plants

Somatic mutations can be detected in petals and stamen hairs in clones heterozygous for flower colour; for example, stamen hairs can develop pink, blue or colourless segments[49] (Figure 6.4).

Tests in insects

The most widely used point mutation test in *Drosophila melanogaster* is that which detects the induction of sex-linked recessive lethals. These become evident in the second generation of treated individuals (Figure 6.5). Such mutations are observed at much lower doses (one-tenth to one five-hundredth) than those needed to induce chromosome loss or dominant lethal mutations in this system. The presence on the X chromosome (which is about 20% of the genome) of many markers makes it possible to classify

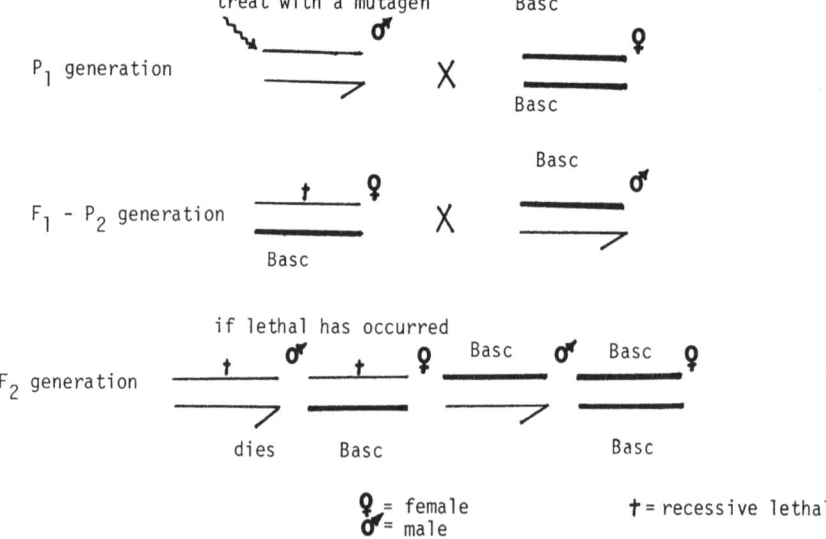

Figure 6.5 Diagram of the sex-linked recessive lethal test when the parental male is treated in *Drosophila melanogaster*. P_1: Wild type males with normal round eyes are treated and mated with virgin Basc females. The Basc chromosome carries the genetic markers Bar and white apricot which give the females narrow-shaped orange eyes. $F_1 - P_2$: The female progeny have kidney-shaped red eyes and have a paternal treated X chromosome which carries a recessive lethal. F_2: The F_2 generation are inspected for the presence of males with round eyes. If this class is missing and has died it can be concluded that the treated male gamete contained a recessive lethal. (The males die because the recessive lethal has no complementary allele on the Y chromosome.

most of the sex-linked recessive lethals as gene mutations or multi-gene deletions. Autosomal recessive lethal mutations can be observed in third generation flies. The induction of visible mutations can be measured by crossing wild males (treated or control) with females homozygous for many visible mutations. The function of *Drosophila* in genetic toxicology testing has been described by Vogel and Sobels[50], Abrahamson and Lewis[51], in various other articles[52-55] and see also Auerbach, chapter 2 in this volume.

Tests in mammalian cells *in vitro*

There are many genetic systems for the detection of point mutations in mammalian cells grown *in vitro*. They are based on the use of phenotypic markers which reveal nutritional, biochemical, serological, temperature sensitivity or antimetabolite resistance; for example Figure 6.6. shows a mutant clone of P388 cells resistant to the antimetabolite 5-iodo-2-deoxyuridine. This antimetabolite blocks the thymidine kinase pathway, consequently, [^{3}H]thymidine is not incorporated in the mutant clone by comparison with wild type cells.

In addition to gene mutation, variants of somatic cells in culture can be generated by phenomenon other than gene mutation, such as gene suppression. Hamster, mouse and human diploid fibroblasts are among the cell lines most often used to detect genetic changes. Some markers are investigated with many cells lines, for example the locus controlling the hypoxanthine guanine phosphoribosyl transferase (HGPRT) enzyme is investigated with Chinese hamster ovary cells[56], Chinese hamster V79 cells[57-64], Chinese hamster lung cells[65], human fibroblast[66] and human lymphoblast cells[67]. The locus controlling adenine phosphoribosyl transferase (APRT) is investigated with human fibroblasts[68]. The thymidine kinase (TK$^+$/$^-$) locus, is investigated with L5178Y[69-71] and P388F mouse lymphoma cells[72-74]. Other markers such as resistance to excess thymidine[72-75], ouabain[75], thioguanine[75,76] and alanine[77] are also investigated with lymphoma cells.

A fluctuation test[78] and a host-mediated assay[79] have also been developed with the L5178Y cells. Attempts have been made to use other mouse lines for mutagenesis assays with a variety of selective agents[80].

Metabolic activation systems

Microbial and mammalian cell systems *in vitro* do not generally possess the metabolic capacity of cells of the intact animal. There are now available

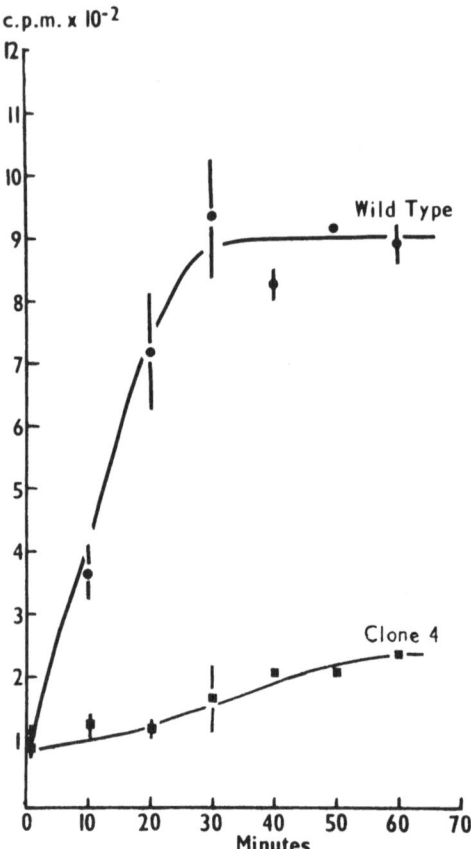

Figure 6.6   Thymidine kinase assay in P388 mouse lymphoma cells and mutant clone measuring [³H]thymidine uptake

systems of metabolic activation such as S-9 mix[2,3,81] which can be used with microbial and mammalian test systems. Figure 6.7 shows a positive response in the P388 mouse lymphoma assay for benzo(a)pyrene in combination with S-9 mix from aroclor-induced and non-induced mouse liver enzymes. Alternatively, feeder layers can be used in combination with mammalian cells in culture. Feeder layers are mammalian cells[82] (usually embryonic with their enzyme systems fully intact) cultivated *in vitro* and inactivated by radiation or a high dose of chemical such as mitomycin C.

In the 'host-mediated assay' (which is relatively insensitive by comparison with the plate incorporation assay since such high doses of test compound have to be used to produce a response) the indicator organism is

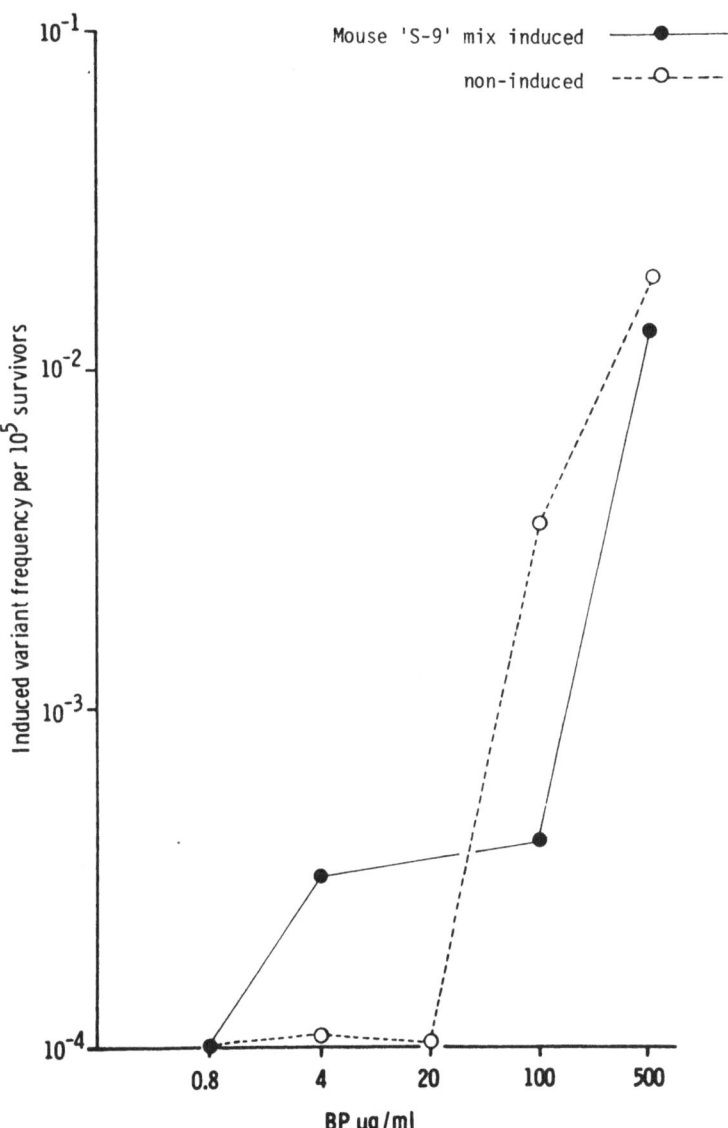

Figure 6.7   P388 Lymphoma cells treated with benzo(a)pyrene

injected into the peritoneal cavity, the circulatory system or the testicles of the host mammal. The animal is then dosed with the substance under test and the indicator organism is recovered from the animal and examined for mutation using an *in vitro* assay. *Salmonella typhimurium*[83], *Escherichia coli*[84], *Saccharomyces cerevisiae*[85,86], *Schizosaccharomyces pombe*, *Neurospora crassa*[83], and mouse lymphoma cells[79], have all been used as indicator organisms.

Chemical substances metabolized by the animal or man may be excreted in the urine[87] as degradation or conjugated products. Microbial indicators can be used to detect mutagenic substances in the urine. Enzymes such as glucuronidase may be used to release the mutagen from its conjugated form[88] (which it might be argued is an unrealistic approach). By analysing the mutagenic activity of the urine or body fluids[89–91] or faeces[92] of human populations it would be possible to screen workers for chemical exposure.

Metabolic activation systems have been described with tests for gene mutation but can also be applied with tests for chromosome damage and DNA repair.

TESTS FOR CHROMOSOME DAMAGE

Chromosome damage is defined as modifications in the number or structure of chromosomes and can be detected both by cytological and genetic methods.

Variations in the number of chromosomes (aneuploidy and polyploidy) may result from endoreduplication (continued chromosome division), metaphase arrest, anaphase retardation and non-disjunction in mitosis and meiosis.

The structural changes are mainly the result of breaks in the chromatid arms. Depending on the number of breaks and the way in which they may join again a whole series of unstable structural modifications may arise which are not transmitted to successive cellular generations, such as 'gaps' (achromatic interruptions), breaks of one or both the chromatids, chromatid interchanges, acentric fragments, ring and dicentric chromosomes. Stable structural modifications which are transmissible may also arise, such as inversions, translocations and deletions. Such changes have been described by Evans[93] and are represented diagrammatically in Figure 6.8.

Tests on micro-organisms

It is possible to measure non-disjunction in micro-organisms. Tests for

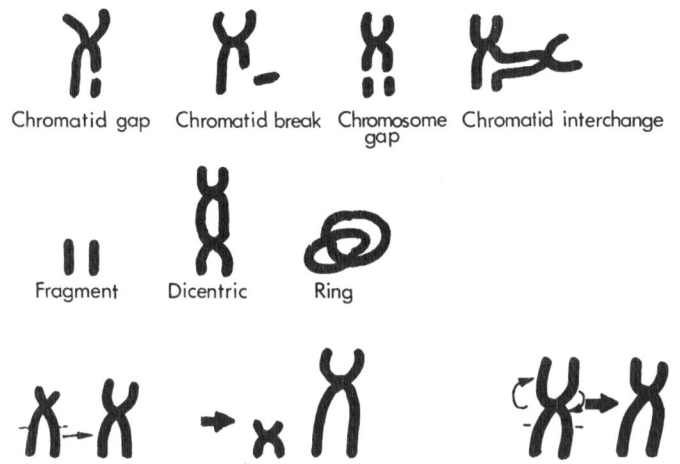

Chromatid gap   Chromatid break   Chromosome   Chromatid interchange
                                        gap

Fragment   Dicentric   Ring

Translocation   Inversion

Figure 6.8   Diagram of different categories of chromosome damage

detecting mitotic non-disjunction have been developed using the fungus *Aspergillus nidulans*[94] and the yeast *Saccharomyces cerevisiae*[95,96], and for measuring meiotic non-disjunction in the fungus *Sordaria brevicollis*[97].

Tests on plants

The radical apices (root tips) of *Vicia faba*[98] (broad bean), *Allium cepa*[98] (common onion) and some species of the genus *Tradescentia*[99] can be used for the detection of chromosome aberrations. However, varying levels of the different categories of chromosome damage have been recorded in onion root tips when compared with Chinese hamster cells[98]. This may be due to differences in the efficiency of the repair system[98]. Consequently such systems may not be suitable for extrapolation to mammalian systems. Chemical mutagenesis in other plants such as *Zea mais* (maize), *Triticum vulgare* (wheat), *Hordeum vulgare* (barley), *Lycopersicum esculentum* (tomato), *Nicotiana tabacum* (tobacco) and *Pisum sativum* (pea) has been reviewed by Ehrenberg[100] and Nilan and Vig[101]. All these plants offer systems for the analysis of chromosomal aberrations.

Tests on insects

Different effects at the chromosome level such as non-disjunction, loss of the X chromosome, deletions, translocations, dominant lethal mutations, mitotic and meiotic recombination can be observed in *Drosophila melano-gaster* as described by Würgler *et al.*[102] and others[51-55]. Changes are generally shown by observing the phenotypes of the progeny from the appropriate crosses; for example reciprocal translocations may be detected in the second generation of treated individuals carrying defined recessive markers in the autosomes. The absence of any of the expected phenotypes in the progeny indicates that translocations occurred in the parent's repro-ductive cells. Also the loss and acquisition of a chromosome or the loss of part of a chromosome can be detected by observing phenotypes in the progeny of crosses in which one of the parents had been treated.

It is also possible cytologically to distinguish chromosome rearrange-ments in the large salivary glands of the generation born from treated flies (Figure 6.9). Somatic recombination is detectable by observing on the

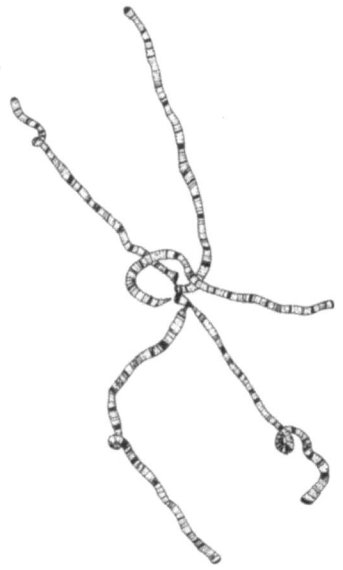

Figure 6.9   Diagram of gland chromosome of *Drosophila melanogaster*. The salivary-gland chromosomes of *Drosophila* show distinct longitudinal differen-tiation, so that particular chromosomes and particular parts of chromosomes are readily identified

adults the twin spots produced by such combination, and meiotic re-combination either by observing the phenotypes or cytological examination of the offspring. The induction of dominant lethals, which are thought to arise from chromosome abnormalities, is determined by comparing the percentage of eggs hatched in crosses between treated and control flies. However, at the genetic level this test cannot distinguish between the effects produced by a compound's toxicity and those due to chromosome abnormalities.

Dominant lethal mutations as measured by hatchability can also be detected using wasps of the genus *Habrobracon*[103,104]. It is possible to distinguish between the transmission of dominant lethal mutations and the loss of fertilizing capacity of the sperm (frequency of fertilized eggs) because of differences in ploidy between the sexes in this insect. The dominant lethal mutations carried by treated individuals' sperms effect only the diploid females, not the haploid males which emerge from parthenogenetic (unfertilized) eggs and the presence of dominant lethals therefore changes the sex ratio (Figure 6.10). With cytotoxic events there is no differential effect. *Bombyx mori* (silkworm) öocytes may also be used for detecting mutagens[105].

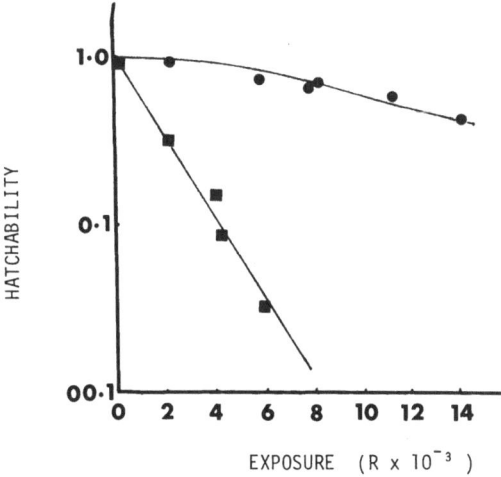

Figure 6.10   Dose-action curves for X-irradiated Habrobracon. Prophase 1 öocytes ● and sperm ■; the öocytes were scored for hatchability of haploid eggs and sperm for hatchability of diploid eggs (data from Von Borstel, R. C. and Rekemeyer, M. L. (1959). *Genetics*, **44**, 1053)

Tests on mammalian cells *in vitro*

Chromosome damage can easily be observed by cytological methods in mammalian cells in culture[93,106]. Human fibroblasts, lymphocytes and

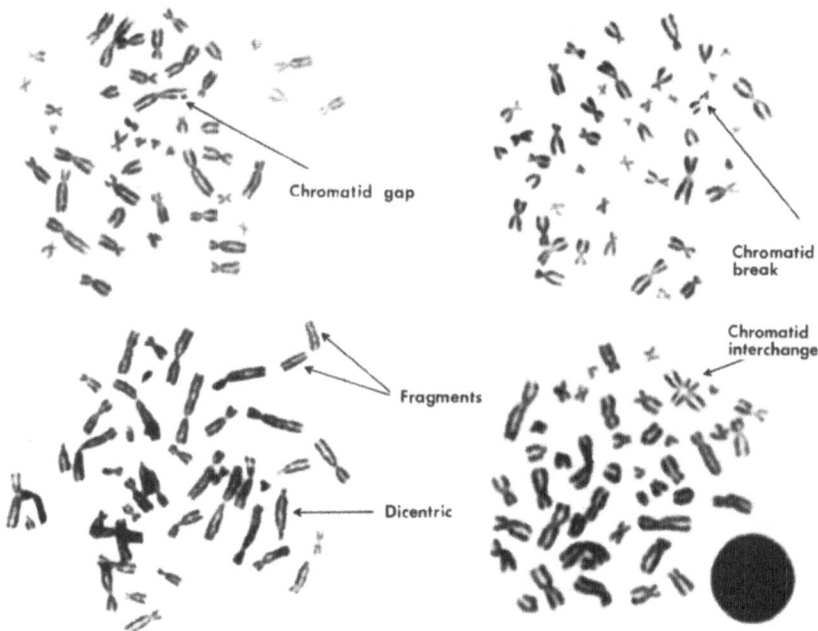

Figure 6.11   Human lymphocytes with different categories of chromosome damage

rodent cells (hamster fibroblasts and mouse lymphocytes) are used. Examples of damage in human lymphocytes is shown in Figure 6.11. Translocations, inversions and other stable rearrangement indicate genetic damage which can be inherited while gaps alone may not indicate such damage but might be indicative of toxic effects. We have carried out considerable work with mutagens in this laboratory on the significance of gaps. We have found them to be associated with chemical mutagenesis and they are a sensitive indicator of a potential mutagen when accompanied by other types of damage (Anderson and Richardson, unpublished). However, we do not yet know whether a toxic non-mutagen can produce gaps in the absence of other categories of chromosome damage.

   The method of sister chromatid exchange in somatic mammalian cells is a measure of the number of crossings-over during replication which occur between identical chromatids following treatment with the test substance[93,107,108] (Figures 6.12, 6.13). It is considered to be a sensitive method for detecting chromosome damage but the significance of the test is not yet fully understood. Such a method is considered as a test which indirectly measures DNA damage involving repair.

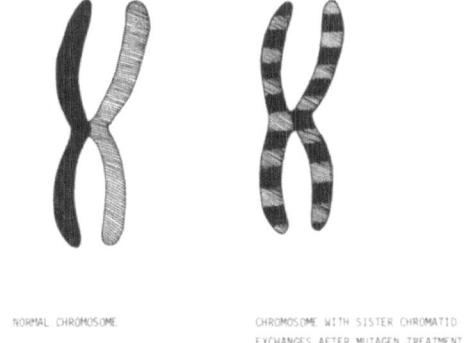

NORMAL CHROMOSOME   CHROMOSOME WITH SISTER CHROMATID
                                     EXCHANGES AFTER MUTAGEN TREATMENT

Figure 6.12   Diagram of sister-chromatid exchanges. To produce the effect represented above the chromosomes replicate twice in medium containing bromodeoxyuridine and are stained with Giemsa (data from Perry, P. and Evans, H. J. (1958). *Nature (London)*, **258**, 121)

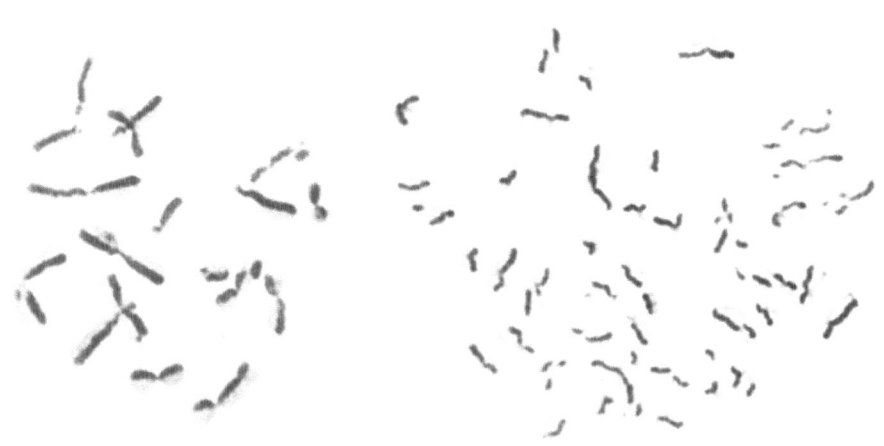

i) In Chinese hamster cells   ii) In human lymphocytes

Figure 6.13   Sister chromatid exchanges

TESTS FOR DNA DAMAGE AND REPAIR

When a chemical reacts with DNA and induces damage, repair normally follows[109,110]. There is excision repair and repair which follows DNA replication known as post-replication repair. These forms of repair are represented diagrammatically in Figures 6.14 and 6.15. Excision repair is

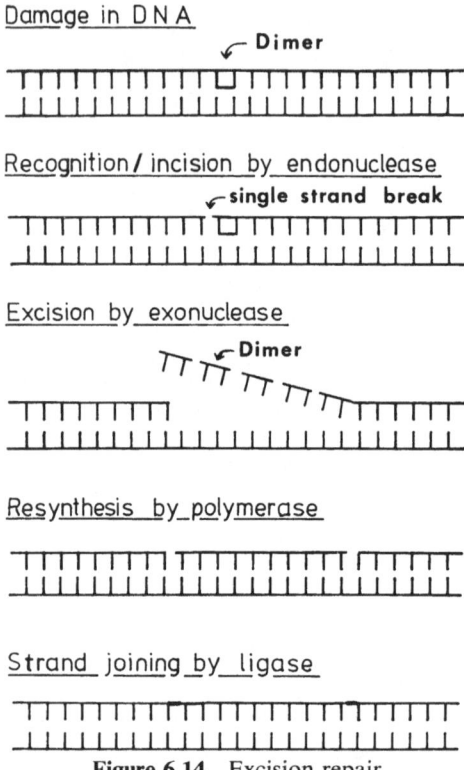

Figure 6.14　Excision repair

an error-free process and post-replication repair is error-prone. The extent of the repair is an indicator of the amount of damage which has occurred to DNA. Damage to the DNA molecule may be considered as a primary lesion which could be involved in the process of development of the mutation (or possibly of formation of neoplastic cells).

Several methods exist for detecting DNA repair phenomenon such as differential zones of inhibition or killing in bacterial strains with and without repair processes[111–114], gene conversion in strains of yeast[39,40], sister chromatid exchanges in mammalian cells[93,107,108] or the direct measurement of DNA damage and repair[109,110].

Tests on micro-organisms

'Spot' tests measuring differential zones of inhibition

A petri dish is seeded or streaked with cells of E. coli,[112] S. typhimurium, Bacillus subtilis[111] and Saccharomyces cerevisiae[40]. The test compound is

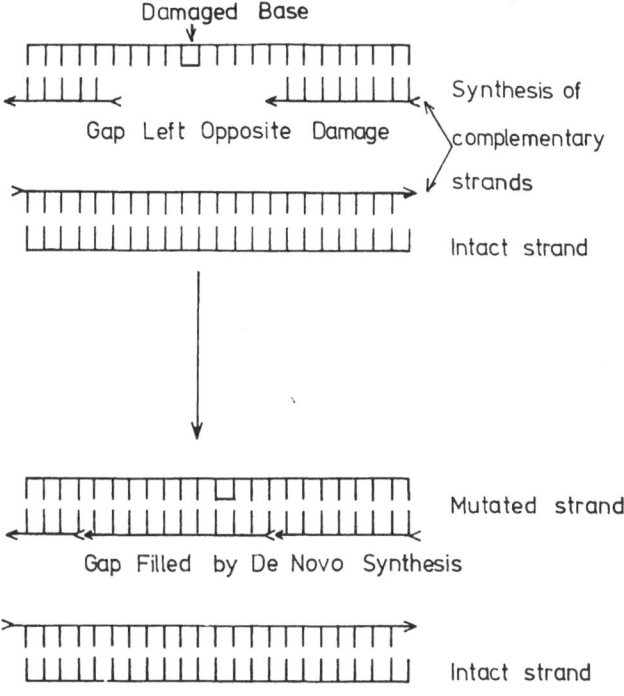

Figure 6.15 Post-replication repair

placed in the dish, and the inhibition zone or lethal effect produced by the compound is evaluated in two different strains of the test organism, one being the wild type strain and the other being deficient in a DNA repair system, such as polA⁻ in *B. subtilis*, rec A⁻ and uvr⁻ in *E. coli*. When a greater zone of inhibition is produced in the repair-deficient strain than in the wild type strain, the compound is considered capable of interfering with DNA and the test shows a positive response (Figure 6.15, (a) compared with (b)). The assay can be carried out with and without metabolic activation (S-9 mix) incorporated in the top agar. If minimal medium is used for the plates as opposed to broth agar, mutation as well as inhibition zones can be detected (Figure 6.16, (c) to (h)). However, such tests are generally considered insensitive[3,31] and recommended for use only as a prescreen.

Tests measuring mitotic recombination or gene conversion

In eukaryotes it is possible to measure an increase in the frequency of mitotic recombination or gene conversion when a recessive phenotype is

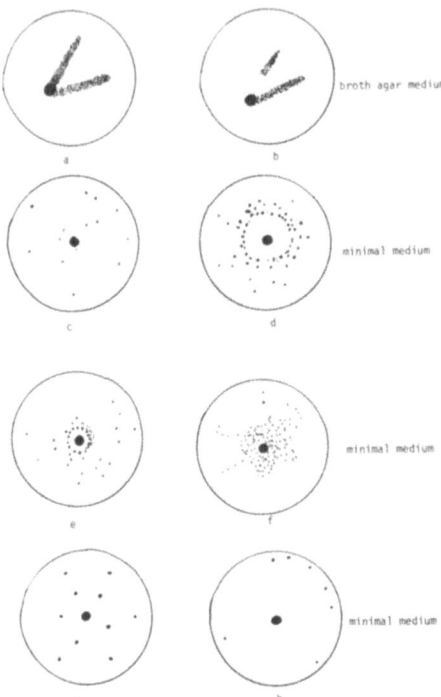

Figure 6.16 Diagram of typical plates from 'spot' tests. (a) Control plate streaked with repair proficient and deficient strains; (b) treated plate streaked with same strains – greater zone of inhibition in repair deficient; (c) control with spontaneous revertants; (d) a positive mutation plate and a zone of inhibition; (e) a positive mutation plate with a smaller zone of inhibition; (f) a positive mutation plate – no zone of inhibition; (g) a zone of inhibition but with no more revertants than in spontaneous control; (h) an intermediate thinning of the lawn around the test disc rather than a distinct zone

expressed in the transition from a heterozyote to a homozygote situation[39,40]. These tests are thought to be related to the exchange following breakage occurring in the chromatids of two homologous chromosomes. Such changes may allow for the expression of recessive mutation since it is known in humans that meiotic recombination allows the expression of recessive gene mutations.

Such tests are carried out in the yeast *Saccharomyces cerevisiae* and *Schizosaccharomyces pombe*[39-42]. A fluctuation test can also be used to detect mitotic gene conversion[44]. Other fungi such as *Aspergillus nidulans* are also used for the same purpose[115].

Tests on mammalian somatic cells in culture

Tests to measure sister chromatid exchange in mammalian cells have already been described on page 110.

Tests to measure DNA repair synthesis

DNA damage can be detected by determining unscheduled DNA synthesis which occurs as a result of DNA excision repair. One of the techniques reveals repair synthesis by determining radioactivity incorporated into DNA as tritiated thymidine during the repair process.

The radioactivity can be measured in two ways either by autoradiography (Figure 6.17) or by direct counting of the incorporated thymidine with a liquid scintillation counter. Metabolic activation can also be included with such systems.

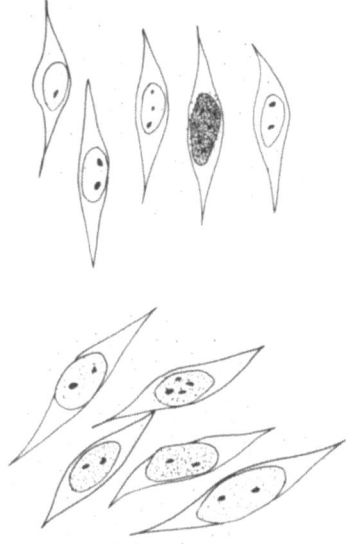

Figure 6.17 Diagram of autoradiograph, representing cultured fibroblasts labelled with [³H]thymidine. Top: control cultures showing one heavily labelled S-phase cell. Bottom: cultures treated with a mutagen showing all lightly labelled repairing cells

Other techniques which can be used to detect chemical action with DNA are the measurement of the breakage of the single DNA chain in alkali,

Table 6.1   Sub-mammalian tests for mutagenesis

Organism	Gene mutation		Chromosome damage[93]*	DNA repair[109,110]
	Forward mutation	*Backward mutation*		
Bacteria	*Salmonella typhimurium* 8-azaguanine resistance[28] Arabinose resistance[29] host-mediated[83] urine and body fluids[87–91] faeces[92] *Escherichia coli* Lack of galactose fermentation[32] 8-methyl-tryptophan resistance[33] Streptomycin resistance[34] induction of prophage[35, 36] fluctuation test[37] host-mediated[84] *Streptomyces coelicolor* Streptomycin resistance[38]	*Salmonella typhimurium* histidine independence[1–8] arginine independence[30] tryptophan independence[31]		*'Spot' tests* *Salmonella typhimurium*[3] *Escherichia coli*[112] *Bacillus subtilis*[111, 114]
Fungi	*Saccharomyces cerevisiae* Adenine dependence[39–42] (also *Schizosaccharomyces pombe*) Canavanine resistance[43] fluctuation test[44] host-mediated[85] *Neurospora crassa* Adenine biosynthesis[45–47] host-mediated[83] *Aspergillus nidulans*[48] 8-azaguanine resistance	methionine independence	*Saccharomyces cerevisiae*[95–96] } mitotic non-disjunction *Aspergillus nidulans*[94] } *Sordaria brevicollis*[97] meiotic non-disjunction	*'Spot' tests* *Saccharomyces cerevisiae*[40] Mitotic gene conversion *Saccharomyces cerevisiae* } 39–42 *Schizosaccharomyces pombe* *Aspergillus nidulons*[115] } 44

Plants	Tradescantia[49] Changes in stamen hairs	Chromosome aberrations Vicia faba[98], Allium cepa[99], Tradescantia[99], other plants[100,101]	
Insects	Drosophila melanogaster Sex-linked recessive lethals } [50-55,102] Autosomal recessive lethals }	Drosophila melanogaster (non-disjunction, dominant lethals, deletions, translocations)[50-55,102] Habrobracon – dominant lethality[103,104] Bombyx mori öocytes[105]	
Mammalian cells in culture	HGPRT locus Chinese hamster ovary[56], V79[57-64], lung cells[65], Human fibroblast cells[66] Human lymphoblast cells[67] Thymidine kinase locus L5178Y cells[69-71] P388F cells[72-74] Excess thymidine[73-75], ouabain[75], thioguanine[75-76], alanine[77] in L5178Y cells L5178Y cells { fluctuation test[78] host-mediated[79] feeder layers[82]	Chromosome aberrations[93,106] Sister-chromatid exchange[107,108]	Sister-chromatid exchange[107-108] Radioactive measurements of repair by autoradiography, liquid scintillation and elution tech- niques[109,110,116]

* NB The numbers refer to the text references.

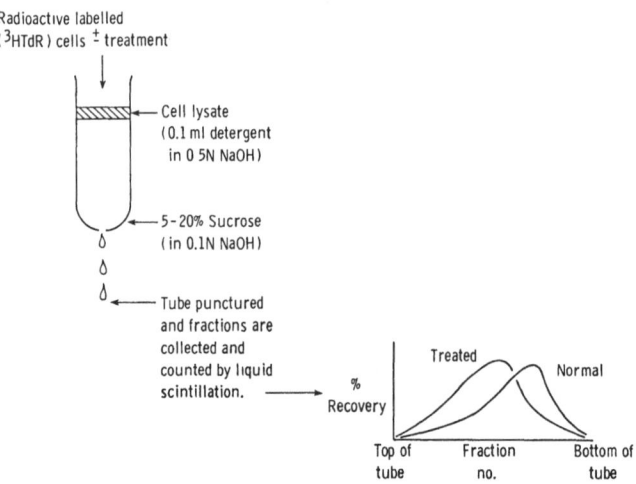

Figure 6.18   Alkaline sucrose gradient sedimentation analysis of DNA

using gradient and elution techniques. The alkaline sucrose gradient sedimentation analysis of DNA is represented diagrammatically in Figure 6.18. The gradient technique is sensitive but the alkaline elution is a simple and faster technique and measures the rate of elution of DNA through a filter. The rate of elution is a function of the DNA's molecular weight. These methods have been described by Cleaver[109,110].

The available tests have therefore been considered according to the three categories; Table 6.1 shows them in summary form together with appropriate text reference numbers. Having considered the three categories, it is seen that there is a wide range of sub-mammalian test systems available for testing compounds but not all of these systems have been equally well studied and some are used by more specialized groups who are not involved in screening chemicals. It is probably true to say that the most widely used test system today is the Ames test. Its widespread use is because of its early validation and subsequent publicity of its potential to detect carcinogens[5,8].

However, this does not mean that other test systems might not be equally useful for detecting carcinogens if sufficient time and effort were spent studying them; for instance other systems such as *Drosophila*[50] and the DNA repair test of Stich[116] have shown similar high correlations with carcinogenicity, but without as many compounds, in several independent laboratories; we have found that *S. typhimurium* can detect mutagen/non-mutagen or carcinogen/non-carcinogen pairs[8,117] but we have also found that *E. coli* is able to differentiate such pairs (Figure 6.19). The drawback

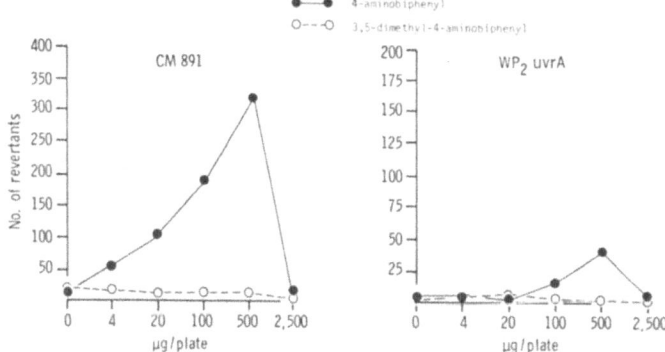

Figure 6.19 *Escherichia coli.* WP₂ uvrA = repair deficient strain; CM 891 = repair deficient strain with plasmid

to using any sub-mammalian system is that extrapolation to mammals is difficult.

SUITABILITY AND USABILITY OF SOME OF THE SYSTEMS FOR SCREENING PURPOSES

Microbial assays

The major advantage of the microbial methods is that they are rapid, cheap and appear to be relatively simple to carry out, but one should never be misled into believing that the tests are simple for the inexperienced worker.

Bacteria

For one person performing tests it has been estimated by Green and Muriel[31] that in *E. coli* over half his time would be spent preparing media, counting experiments, tabulating data, etc., leaving about 3 hours per day only to carry out experiments. (However, for large-scale testing, suppliers are available from whom poured plates can be bought (Difco and Gibco Biocult) and colony counters which reduce the burden of counting plates). In the 3 hours about 15 spot-tests could be carried out, with treat and plate method, about six survival or mutation curves of three points can be performed in a similar period, and fluctuation test with two tests of three concentrations of compound plus a control can be performed. Allowing for repetition and difficulties, in these three methods these values can be corrected to two compounds per person per day in the first system and one compound per person per 9 days in the other two systems. These estimates would be similar for other bacterial systems. Bacteria allow for detection of both gene mutation and DNA repair.

Yeasts

Both *Saccharomyces cerevisiae* and *Schizosaccharomyces pombe* are suitable for use in routine screening assays[40]. Strains can be cultivated in the diploid as well as in the haploid phase and this allows for the detection of a wide spectrum of mutational events. Yeasts can be used to detect both point mutations and DNA repair events in terms of mitotic recombination as evaluated by crossing-over and gene conversion. One disadvantage is that the chromosomes are too small for direct cytological observation but chromosome damage can be measured by tests for non-disjunction. Yeast systems take a few days longer than bacterial systems for colony growth but the overall time-scale involved is not greatly different.

Plant systems

Plant systems can detect most types of damage. They have short generation times, the cost, handling and space requirements are relatively small; the cost and time training a technician to handle a variety of endpoints following mutagen treatment is relatively small; genetics of seeds can be investigated under a wide range of environmental conditions such as pH, water content, temperature; and chromosome organization is similar to the human system, etc.[101] Difficulty is experienced, however, in relating actions in plants, since the knowledge obtained from plants may not be directly transferable to man either quantitatively or even qualitatively. Several agents like cytosine-arabinoside, daunomycin and adriamycin are known to be ineffective on the plant genomes in spite of severe genetic damage caused by these chemicals in mammalian cells. This is possibly because the cell wall which surrounds a plant cell has an influence on the penetration of a compound into the cell and because of the suspected differences in repair between plant and animal cells[98]. Such systems are therefore probably not satisfactory for predicting potential human mutagens.

Insect systems

Drosophila has a short generation time of 10–12 days, is cheap and easy to breed in large numbers with relatively simple facilities. Extensive studies on the metabolism of insecticides performed during the last 15 years[102] have revealed that insect microsomes are capable of facilitating similar enzymic reactions to those from the mammalian liver, but insects do not have any specific organ in which those enzymes are predominantly located. The nature and diversity of the reactions catalysed indicate that insect microsomes exhibit a similar degree of metabolic versatility and substrate non-specificity as those from the mammalian liver. In *Drosophila* mutagenic activity can be tested in a wide variety of different germ cell stages. This is important because some mutagens have specificity of action. *Drosophila* permits the scoring for the whole spectrum of genetic effects. The observation that the lowest effective concentration (LEC) values and thus the highest mutagenic effectiveness has been recorded for recessive lethals clearly indicate the superior descriminating power of this test, and since the X chromosome represents a fifth of the small number of *Drosophila* chromosomes a test for recessive lethals samples a significant section of the whole genome. By comparison the test for dominant lethality is of limited value because high doses are required to produce effects, and dominant lethals sometimes fail to arise with agents which cause the induction of recessive lethals and spurious changes in hatchability sometimes produce false-positives. However, *Drosophila* is a good 'catch-all' system due to the variety of genetic endpoints which can be detected. It has been estimated by Wurgler et al.[102] that with two technicians and one laboratory helper, two experiments consisting of three successive broods each can be handled per week per compound to detect recessive lethal mutations together with a dominant lethal or a chromosome loss test. It is estimated that the total annual capacity with the above staff is about 40 compounds a year but with one technician it would be more realistically six compounds a year.

Mammalian systems

Mammalian cell systems are generally considered more valid than non-mammalian systems in terms of extrapolation to man in that mammalian DNA is more similar to that of man. Whilst normal diploid human cells are obviously desirable for mutation assays they are more difficult to handle from a screening viewpoint than malignant cells in culture due to their low plating efficiencies and lack of perpetual proliferation. Lymphoma cells which grow in suspension are even easier to handle than cells which grow as a monolayer. They do not require trypsinization, are very easily subcultured and they are not subject to metabolic co-operation. Where cells metabolically co-operate mutation frequencies can be lowered when mutagenic cells are in close contact with non-mutagenic cells.

The test systems measuring mutation can take varying lengths of time to test a compound. The exact length of time can depend on the marker investigated and the cell system used. There are varying expression times before different mutations are expressed. A survival assay can be performed beforehand to determine the correct survival range. One person can test about one compound over five doses per 2 months allowing for repetition and difficulties.

DNA repair tests

The question is often asked whether DNA repair has any significance for the mutagenic potential of a chemical. This is important because measurements of excision repair are averages over all the cells in a population, whereas mutation is a rare event in individual cells. The amount of excision repair after exposure to an agent will depend on several factors according to Cleaver[109]. These are the extent of reaction with the DNA, that is, the total number of damaged sites, the number of sites which can be excision repaired, the size of the repaired regions, the kinetics of excision repair as functions of time and dose and the extent to which chemical interactions modify other sites, particularly in proteins, and possibly inhibit excision repair. The amount of excision repair will therefore be greatest for mutagens that induce the greatest proportion of damaged sites that are repairable by the larger patches. The number of mutations will depend on different factors, especially the amount of unrepaired or irreparable damage that is in DNA at the time of DNA replication and the probability that during post-replication, repair of this damage will induce mutations of any kind such as point mutations, frameshifts, deletions or insertions. Studies of the relationship between DNA damage, excision repair, post-replication repair and mutagenesis must take into account the numbers and varieties of lesions involved in mutagenesis and their modes of repair. Exclusive reliance on any one measurement is not satisfactory since it is difficult to predict the amount of unrepaired damage from excision repair measurements. Thus it is best to consider DNA repair only in conjunction with some other parameter before assessing the possible mutagenicity of an agent. Tests for DNA repair will vary in the length of time to carry out the study depending on the technique used. The method of autoradiography generally takes longer than elution techniques.

SIGNIFICANCE AND INTERPRETATION OF THE TESTS

Most of the available sub-mammalian test systems have been considered. It should be pointed out that at present these test systems used without mammalian *in vivo* studies would not be acceptable by any governmental authority for estimating risk evaluation to man. However, they do provide a useful tool for a preliminary screening of potential human mutagens. A positive result exhibiting a dose–response in the more well-validated systems is generally regarded as a warning sign. However, when assessing chemicals of unknown mutagenic potential it must be remembered that most of the classic dose–response effects reported in the mutagenicity literature are based on experiments repeated and refined using radiation and powerful alkylating agents (which are often 'radiomimetic'). The transition from this situation to the real world of screening many diverse chemicals, most of which require metabolic activation and may react differently with different cells and organs before producing genotoxic effects, is a difficult one. It is therefore, not surprising that many of the environmental chemicals which have recently been evaluated give equivocal data which cannot be resolved from experience gained from classical studies.

Results are not always clearly defined for compounds of unknown mutagenic potential and various problems can arise in interpretation of data; for example, assuming that results are reproducible in well-conducted experiments using adequate testing protocols, interpretation of data may be difficult especially when results are near the control range and on the borderline of statistical significance. Interpretation may differ depending on whether results from treatment groups are compared with historical (accumulated) or concurrent controls, the type of statistical analysis employed and whether results are compared at equitoxic doses. If doubtful experiments are repeated, similar equivocal results may be obtained and if not there is the problem of whether the first or repeat experiment is correct. The difficulty is in proving and accepting negative data.

By comparison, the handling of positive data is much more clear-cut for it is relatively easy to establish the genetic activity of an agent. This is particularly so where activity leads to an absolute increase in the number of mutants per treated cell, because the rate of increase of mutants over spontaneous is greater than the rate of inactivation, per unit dose increase. Weak mutagens, however, are difficult to evaluate because sometimes there is only an increase in mutants per surviving cell (that is, after correction for survival) but not per treated cell. The observed relative increase may be due to the induction of new mutants or it may be due to a higher resistance of spontaneous mutants to the inactivating effects of the agent used. Reconstruction experiments can solve the former problem but to the latter there is no good solution. It is desirable that dose–response curves should be established in routine testing. However, difficulties may arise since some mutagens induce high frequencies of genetic alterations long

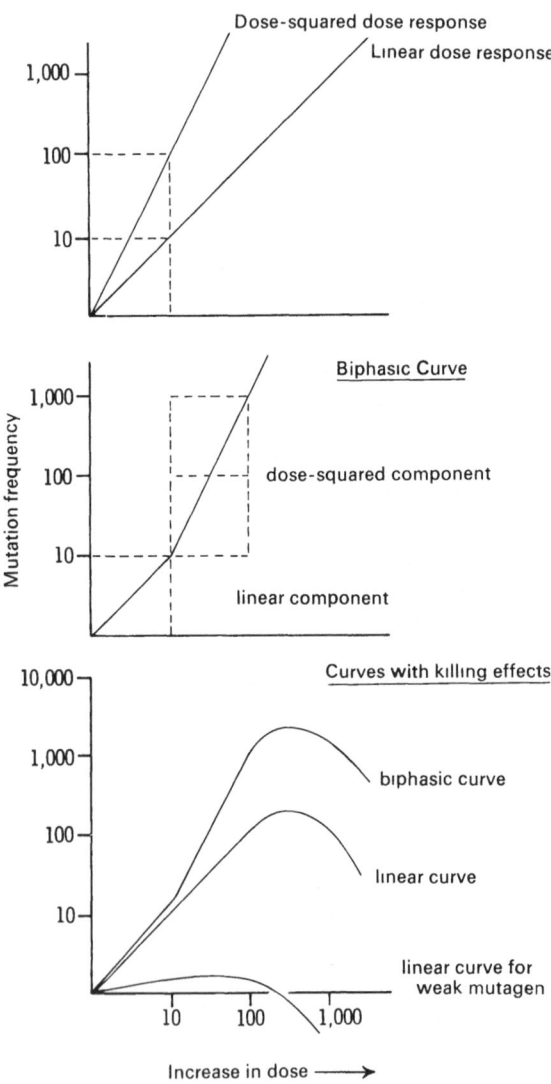

Figure 6.20 Dose-response curves

before killing becomes significant whilst other mutagens have a strong killing effect and exhibit less genetic activity; so in the latter case, a genetic effect is obviously not as readily detected. Dose–response curves generally have linear (single 'hit') and dose-squared (two 'hit') kinetics and may be biphasic with a linear function at low doses and a dose-squared component at higher doses. Thresholds may even exist at some chemical concentrations. At higher doses, response curves can plateau and even decline when the killing effect is strong (Figure 6.20). When dose–response curves are present it is easier to reach a conclusion on the mutagenicity of a chemical, but if a wide enough dose range has been used a single optimal dose, or the dose which gives the highest mutation frequency, can be used as a basis for comparison of its mutagenicity.

CONCLUSIONS

The main problem with the present methods of testing for mutagenicity is that not all systems are equally reliable and reproducible. (The current international evaluation of short-term tests may elucidate this problem.) Even the systems in which most compounds have been tested such as the Ames test, give different results for some compounds in some laboratories. Ideally, a system for monitoring chemicals for mutagenic activity should (1) detect the potential of the test substance to induce gene and chromosome mutations in somatic or germ cells, (2) provide quantitative data for extrapolation to man, (3) be capable of detecting metabolic products of the compound which have mutagenic potential, (4) be reliable and reproducible, (5) be economically viable and quick. Unfortunately however, no one test system at present meets all these demands.

A combination of tests is required. For example, if a single bacterial system which detects gene mutation is used and a substance does not cause gene mutation but does cause chromosome damage (such as benzene) then a compound's mutagenic potential would not be realized. Such a battery should preferentially consist of a microbial test plus a chromosome damaging test and this combination would be the minimum of tests required. If a larger battery were to be used then it is not really worth carrying out more than one prokaryotic bacterial assay unless different end-points are to be examined or if it is known that another prokaryotic assay will detect a class of compounds which the first prokaryotic assay does not. It would be better to consider a eukaryotic cell system to identify those which are potentially hazardous to man. Plant systems may be too misleading for this purpose but a fungal cell system, *Drosophila*, or a mammalian cell system might be more useful. It should be pointed out, however, that by making the test battery too large a greater number of false results may be generated. This has been considered by Purchase et al.[117]. It is suggested that the 'gap' which is thought to exist between mutagenicity and carcinogenicity may be partially bridged at an early stage of testing with a cell transformation assay, such as that of Styles, which appears to respond equally well to carcinogens and mutagens[117].

Both industrial and academic scientists are well aware of the need for safety evaluation in general toxicological testing and this is certainly true in the field of genetic toxicology. Two review articles highlight this awareness[26,118]. However, we are still not always certain if positive or negative results in laboratory model test systems are relevant to man because of man's unique metabolism and because of the absence of any convincing 'no-effect' level data for animals and man. However, we do have thousands of untested chemicals in our environment and some attempt should be made to identify those which are potentially hazardous to man. The limitations of the simple short-term tests which are more concerned with the concept of somatic mutation than of heritable genetic damage, are becoming better understood and the problems of false-positives and negative results are now being considered. To extrapolate to man in terms of heritable damage, in vivo animal studies are really required. Tests for this purpose however, such as the specific locus test[119,120] and heritable translocation test[121,122] require very large numbers of animals, extensive housing and maintenance and do not necessarily generate sufficient information to assess the genetic risk to man. There is a current school of opinion which holds that since mutagenicity tests detect carcinogens, carcinogenicity tests may equally well detect mutagens. This opinion is based on the concept that cancer may be an easily observable phenotype of DNA mutation. If this is so then the carcinogenicity and mutagenicity data for a chemical should be considered together and not as disparate phenomena.

References

1. Ames, B. N., Lee, F. D. and Durston, W. E. (1973). An improved bacterial test system for the detection and classification of mutagens and carcinogens. Proc. Natl. Acad. Sci. (USA), 70, 782
2. Ames, B. N., Durston, W. E., Yamaski, E. and Lee, F. D. (1973). Carcinogens are mutagens: a simple test system combining liver homogenates for activation and bacteria for detection. Proc. Natl. Acad. Sci. (USA), 70, 2281
3. Ames, B. N., McCann, J. and Yamasaki, E. (1975). Methods for detecting carcinogens and mutagens with the Salmonella/mammalian microsome mutagenicity test. Mutation Res., 31, 347
4. McCann, J., Spingarn, N. E., Kobori, J. and Ames, B. N. (1975). The

detection of carcinogens as mutagens: bacterial tester strains with R factor plasmids. *Proc. Natl. Acad. Sci. (USA)*, **72**, 979
5. McCann, J., Choi, E., Yamasaki, E. and Ames, B. N. (1975). Detection of carcinogens as mutagens in the *Salmonella*/microsome test. Part I, Assay of 300 chemicals. *Proc. Natl. Acad. Sci. (USA)*, **72**, 5135
6. McCann, J. and Ames, B. N. (1976). Detection of carcinogens as mutagens in the *Salmonella*/microsome test. Assay of 300 chemicals. Part II. *Proc. Natl. Acad. Sci. (USA)*, **73**, 950
7. Coombs, M. M., Dixon, C. and Kissonerghis, A. M. (1976). Evaluation of the mutagenicity of compounds of known carcinogenicity belonging to the benz[a]anthracene, chrysene and cyclopenta[a]phenanthrene series, using Ames' test. *Cancer Res.*, **36**, 4525
8. Purchase, I. F. H., Longstaff, E., Ashby, J., Styles, J. A., Anderson, D., Lefevre, P. A. and Westwood, F. R. (1976). Evaluation of six short-term tests for detecting organic chemical carcinogens and recommendations for their use. *Nature (London)*, **264**, 624
9. Joint FAO/WHO 1961. Expert Committee on Food Additives: Evaluation of the carcinogenic hazards of food additives. *WHO Tech. Rep. Ser.*, No. 220
10. Carter, C. O. (1977). The relative contribution of mutant genes and chromosome abnormalities to genetic ill-health in man. In: D. Scott, B. A. Bridges and F. H. Sobels (eds.). *Progress in Genetic Toxicology* pp. 1–14. (Amsterdam: Elsevier Biomedical Press, North-Holland.)
11. McKusick, V. (1971). *Mendelian Inheritance in Man*. 3rd ed. (Baltimore: Johns Hopkins Press.)
12. Bochkov, N. P., Srám, R. J., Kulehsov, N. P. and Zhurkov, V. S. (1975). Test systems for evaluation of mutagenic activity of chemicals in man: general principles, practical recommendations and further elaboration. *Genetika*, **11**, 156
13. Legator, M. S. and Malling, H. V. (1969). Concepts in animal testing for chemical mutagens. *Genetics*, **61**, S5
14. Vogel, F. and Röhrborn, G. (1970). Concluding remarks. In: E. Vogel and G. Röhrborn (eds.). *Chemical mutagenesis in Mammals and Man*, pp. 453–459 (Berlin, Heidelberg and New York: Springer-Verlag)
15. Advisory Committee on Protocols for Safety Evaluation (1970). Panel on reproduction, report on reproduction studies in the safety evaluation of food additives and pesticide residues. *Toxicol. Appl. Pharmacol.*, **16**, 264
16. WHO Report (1971). The evaluation and testing of drugs for mutagenicity principles and problems. *WHO Tech. Rep. Ser.*, No. 482
17. WHO Report (1974). Assessment of the carcinogenicity and mutagenicity of chemicals. *WHO Tech. Rep. Ser.*, No. 546
18. WHO Report (1975). Guidelines for evaluation of drugs for use in man. *WHO Tech. Rep. Ser.*, No. 563
19. Evaluation of genetic risks of environmental chemicals (1973). (Stockholm: Royal Swedish Academy of Sciences), Ambio Special Report No. 31
20. The testing of chemicals for carcinogenicity, mutagenicity and teratogenicity (1973). *Hlth and Welfare*, Ottawa, Canada
21. Bridges, B. A. (1973). Some general principles of mutagenicity screening and a possible framework for testing procedure. *Environ. Hlth Perspect.*, No. 6, 221

22. Bridges, B. A. (1974). The three-tier approach to mutagenicity screening and the concept of the radiation-equivalent dose. *Mutat. Res.*, **26**, 335
23. Matter, B. E. (1976). Problems of testing drugs for potential mutagenicity. *Mutat. Res.*, **38**, 243
24. Flamm, W. G. (1974). A tier approach to mutagen testing. *Mutat. Res.*, **24**, 329
25. Committee 17 (1975). Environmental mutagenic hazards: Mutagenicity screening is now feasible and necessary for chemicals entering the environment. *Science*, **187**, 503
26. Anderson, D. (1968). An appraisal of the current state of mutagenicity testing. *J. Soc. Cosmet. Chem.*, **29**, 207
27. Ashby, J. and Styles, J. A. (1978). Does carcinogenic potency correlate with mutagenic potency in the Ames' assay? *Nature (London)*, **271**, 452; **274**, 19
28. Skopek, T. R., Liber, J. L., Krowleski, J. J. and Thilly, W. G. (1978). Quantitative forward mutation assay in *Salmonella typhimurium* using 8-azaguanine resistance as a genetic marker. *Proc. Natl. Acad. Sci. (USA)*, **75**, 410
29. Pueyo, C. (1978). A forward mutation assay using a 1-arabinose sensitive strain. Abstracts (Ab^{-2}). *American Environmental Mutagen Society*
30. Mohn, G., Ellenberger, J. and McGregor, D. B. (1974). Development of mutagenicity tests using *Escherichia coli* K-12 as an indicator organism. *Mutat. Res.*, **23**, 187
31. Green, M. H. L. and Muriel, W. J. (1976). Mutagen testing using tryp$^+$ reversion in *Escherichia coli*. *Mutat. Res.*, **38**, 3
32. Saedler, H., Gullon, A., Fiethen, L. and Starlinger, P. (1968). Negative control of the galactose operon in *Escherichia coli*. *Mol. Gen. Genet.*, **102**, 79
33. Mohn, G. (1973). 5-methyl-tryptophan resistance mutations in *Escherichia coli* K-12. Mutagenic activity of monofunctional alkylating agents including organophosphorus insecticides. *Mutat. Res.*, **20**, 7
34. Wild, D. (1973). Chemical induction of streptomycin-resistant mutations in *Escherichia coli*. Dose and mutagenic effects of dichlorvos and methylmethanesulphonate. *Mutat. Res.*, **19**, 33
35. Moreau, P., Bailone, A., Devoret, R. (1976). Prophage induction in *Escherichia coli* K-12 envA uvrB: a highly sensitive test for potential carcinogens. *Proc. Natl. Acad. Sci. (USA)*, **73**, 3700
36. Speck, W. T., Santella, R. M. and Rozenkranz, H. S. (1978). An evaluation of the prophage induction (inductest) for the detection of potential carcinogens. *Mutat. Res.*, **54**, 101
37. Green, M. H. L., Muriel, W. J. and Bridges, B. A. (1976). Use of a simplified fluctuation test to detect low levels of mutagens. *Mutat. Res.*, **38**, 33
38. Carere, A., Morpurgo, G., Cardamone, G., Bignami, M., Aulicino, F., Di Guisepie G., and Conti, C. (1975). Point mutations induced by pharmaceutical drugs. *Mutat. Res.*, **29**, 235
39. Mortimer, R. K. and Manney, T. R. (1971). Mutation induction in yeast. In: A. Hollaender (ed.). *Chemical Mutagens, Principles and Methods for their Detection, Vol. 1*, pp. 209–237. (New York, London: Plenum Press)
40. Zimmerman, F. K. (1973). Detection of genetically active chemicals using

various yeast systems. In: A. Hollaender (ed.). *Chemical Mutagens, Principles and Methods for their Detection Vol. 3*, pp. 209–237. (New York, London: Plenum Press)

41. Zimmerman, F. K. (1975). Procedures used in the induction of mitotic recombination and mutation in the yeast *Saccharomyces cerevisiae*. *Mutat. Res.*, **31**, 71

42. Loprieno, N., Barale, R., Bauer, C., Baroncelli, S., Bronzetti, G., Cammellini, A., Cinci, A., Corsi, G., Leporini, C., Nieri, R., Mozzolini, M. and Serra, C. (1974). The use of different test systems with yeasts for the evaluation of chemically induced gene conversions and gene mutations. *Mutat. Res.*, **25**, 197

43. Brusick, D. J. (1972). Induction of cyclohexamide resistant mutants in *Saccharomyces cerevisiae* with N-methyl-N-nitro-N-nitrosoguanidine and ICR-170. *J. Bacteriol.*, **109**, 1134

44. Parry, J. M. (1977). The use of yeast cultures for the detection of environmental mutagens using a fluctuation test. *Mutat. Res.*, **46**, 165

45. Ong, T. M., de Serres, F. J. (1972). Mutagenicity of chemical carcinogens in *Neurospora crassa*. *Cancer Res.*, **32**, 1890

46. De Serres, F. J. and Malling, H. V. (1971). Measurement of recessive lethal damage over the entire genome and at two specific loci in the ad-3 region of a two component heterokaryon of *Neurospora crassa*. In: A. Hollaender (ed.). *Chemical Mutagens, Principles and Methods for their Detection, Vol. 2*, pp. 311–341 (New York, London: Plenum Press)

47. Ong, T. M. (1978). Use of the spot, plate and suspension test systems for the detection of the mutagenicity of environmental agents and chemical carcinogens in *Neurospora crassa*. (In press)

48. Roper, J. A. (1971) *Aspergillus*. In: A. Hollaender (ed.). *Chemical Mutagens, Principles and Methods for their Detection Vol. 2*, pp. 343–365. (New York, London: Plenum Press)

49. Underbrink, A. G., Schairer, L. A. and Sparrow, A. H. (1973). *Tradescantia* stamen hairs. A radiobiological test system applicable to chemical mutagenesis. In: A. Hollaender (ed.). *Chemical Mutagens, Principles and Methods for their Detection, Vol. 3*, pp. 171–207. (New York, London: Plenum Press)

50. Vögel, E. and Sobels, F. H. (1976). The function of *Drosophila* in genetic toxicology testing. In: A. Hollaender (ed.). *Chemical Mutagens, Principles and Methods for their Detection, Vol. 4*, pp. 93–132. (New York, London: Plenum Press)

51. Abrahamson, S. and Lewis, E. B. (1971). The detection of mutations in *Drosophila*. In: A. Hollaender (ed.). *Chemical Mutagens, Principles and Methods for their Detection, Vol. 2*, pp. 461–489 (New York, London: Plenum Press)

52. Mollet, P., Würgler, F. E. (1974). Detection of somatic recombination and mutation in *Drosophila*. A method for testing genetic activity of chemical compounds. *Mutat. Res.*, **25**, 421

53. Mollet, P., Weilenmann, W. (1976). Characteristics of a new mutagenicity test: induction of somatic recombination and mutation in *Drosophila* by different chemicals. *Mutat. Res.*, **38**, 131

54. Vogel, E. (1977). Identification of carcinogens by mutagen testing in

Drosophila: the relative reliability for the kinds of genetic damage measured. In: H. H. Hiatt, J. D. Watson and J. A. Winston (eds.). *Origins of Human Cancer, Vol. C*, pp. 1483–1497. (New York: Cold Spring Harbor Laboratory)

55. Baker, B. S., Boyd, J. B., Carpenter, A. T. C., Green, M. M., Nguyen, T. D., Ripoll, P. and Smith, P. D. (1976). Genetic controls of meiotic recombination and somatic DNA metabolism in *Drosophila melanogaster*. *Proc. Natl. Acad. Sci. (USA)*, **73**, 4140

56. Neill, J. P., Brimer, P. A., Machanoff, R., Hirsch, G. P. and Hsie, A. W. (1977). A quantitative assay of mutation induction at the HGPRT locus in Chinese hamster ovary cells: development and definition of the system. *Mutat. Res.*, **45**, 91

57. Huberman, E. and Sachs, L. (1974). Cell-mediated mutagenesis of mammalian cells with chemical carcinogens. *Int. J. Cancer*, **13**, 326

58. Krahn, D. F. and Heidelberger, C. (1977). Liver homogenate-mediated mutagenesis in Chinese hamster V79 cells by polycyclic 'aromatic' hydrocarbons and aflatoxins. *Mutat. Res.*, **46**, 27

59. Chu, E. H. Y., Brimer, P., Jacobson, K. B. and Merriam, E. V. (1976). Mammalian cell genetics 1. Selection and characterization of mutations auxotrophic for 1-glutamine or resistance to 8-azaguanine in Chinese hamster cells *in vitro*. *Genetics*, **62**, 359

60. Fox, M., Boyle, J. M. and Fox, B. W. (1976). Biological and biochemical characteristics of purine analogue resistant clones of V79 Chinese hamster cells. *Mutat. Res.*, **25**, 219

61. Nikaido, O. and Fox, M. (1976). The relative effectiveness of 6-thioguanine and 8-azaguanine in selecting resistant mutants from two V79 Chinese hamster clones *in vitro*. *Mutat. Res.*, **35**, 279

62. Arlett, C. F. (1977). Mutagenicity testing with V79 Chinese hamster cells. In: B. J. Kilbey, M. Legator, W. Nichols and C. Ramel (eds.). *Handbook of Mutagenicity Test Procedures*, pp. 175–191. (Amsterdam: Elsevier Biomedical Press, North-Holland)

63. Duncan, R. E. and Brooks, P. (1974). Enzyme activities in extracts of 8-azaguanine resistant mutants of cultured Chinese hamster cells induced by the carcinogen 7-bromomethyl benz[a]anthracene. *Mutat. Res.*, **26**, 37

64. Gillin, F. D., Roufa, D. J., Beaudet, A. L. and Caskey, C. T. (1972). 8-azaguanine resistance in mammalian cells. 1-hypoxanthine guanine phosphoribosyl transferase. *Genetics*, **72**, 239

65. Dean, B. J. and Senner, K. R. (1977). Detection of chemically induced mutation in Chinese hamsters. *Mutat. Res.* **46**, 403

66. Jacobs, L. and De Mars, R. (1977). Chemical mutagenesis with diploid human fibroblasts. In: B. J. Kilbey, M. Legator, W. Nichols and C. Ramel (eds.). *Handbook of Mutagenicity Test Procedures*, pp. 193–220. (Amsterdam: Elsevier Biomedical Press, North-Holland)

67. Thilly, W. G., De Luca, J. G., Hoppe, I. V. H., Penmann, B. W. (1976). Mutation of human lymphoblasts by methyl nitrosourea. *Chem. Biol. Interact.*, **15**, 33

68. De Mars, R. (1974). Resistance of cultured human fibroblasts and other cells to purine and pyrimidine analogues in relation to mutagenesis detection. *Mutat. Res.*, **24**, 335

69. Clive, D. W. and Spector, J. F. S. (1975). Laboratory procedure for assessing specific locus mutations at the TK locus in cultured L5178Y mouse lymphoma cells. *Mutat. Res.*, **31**, 17
70. Clive, D. W. (1973). Recent developments with the L5178Y TK heterozygote mutagen assay system. *Environ. Hlth Perspect.*, No. **6**, 119
71. Clive, D. W., Flamm, W. G., Machesko, M. R. and Bernheim, N. H. (1972). Mutational assay system using the thymidine kinase locus in mouse lymphoma cells. *Mutat. Res.*, **16**, 77
72. Anderson, D. and Fox, M. (1974). The induction of thymidine and IUdR resistant variants in P388 mouse lymphoma cells by X-rays, UV and mono- and bifunctional alkylating agents. *Mutat. Res.*, **25**, 107
73. Anderson, D. (1975). The selection and induction of 5-iodo-2-deoxyuridine and thymidine variants of P388 mouse lymphoma cells with agents which are used for selection. *Mutat. Res.*, **33**, 399
74. Fox, M. and Anderson, D. (1974). Induced thymidine and 5-iodo-2-deoxyuridine resistant clones of mouse lymphoma cells. *Mutat. Res.*, **25**, 89
75. Cole, J. and Arlett, C. F. (1976). Ethyl methanesulphonate mutagenesis with L5178Y mouse lymphoma cells. A comparison of ouabain, thioguanine and excess thymidine resistance. *Mutat. Res.*, **34**, 507
76. Knaap, A. G. A. C. and Simons, J. W. I. M. (1975). A mutational assay system for L5178Y mouse lymphoma cells using hypoxanthine guanine phosphoribosyl transferase deficiency as a marker. The occurrence of a long expression time for mutations induced by X-rays and EMS. *Mutat. Res.*, **30**, 97
77. Nakamura, J., Suzuki, N. and Okada, S. (1977). Mutagenicity of furylfuramide, a food preservative tested by using alanine – requiring mouse L5178Y cells *in vitro* and *in vivo*. *Mutat. Res.*, **46**, 355
78. Cole, J., Arlett, C. F. and Green, M. H. L. (1976). The fluctuation test as a more sensitive system for determining induced mutation in L5178Y mouse lymphoma cells. *Mutat. Res.*, **41**, 377
79. Fischer, G. A., Lee, S. Y. and Calabresi, P. (1974). Detection of chemical mutagens using a host-mediated assay L5178Y mutagenesis system. *Mutat. Res.*, **26**, 501
80. Anderson, D. (1975). Attempts to produce systems for isolating spontaneous and induced variants in various mouse lymphoma cells using a variety of selective agents. *Mutat. Res.*, **33**, 407
81. Frantz, C. N. and Malling, H. V. (1975). The quantitative microsomal mutagenesis assay method. *Mutat. Res.*, **31**, 365
82. Huberman, E. (1975). Mammalian cell transformation and cell-mediated mutagenesis by carcinogenic polycyclic hydrocarbons. *Mutat. Res.*, **29**, 285
83. Legator, M. S. and Malling, H. V. (1971). The host-mediated assay, a practical procedure for evaluating potential mutagenic agents in mammals. In: A. Hollaender (ed.). *Chemical Mutagens, Principles and Methods for their Detection, Vol. 2*, pp. 569–589. (New York and London: Plenum Press)
84. Mohn, G. and Ellenberger, J. (1973). Mammalian blood-mediated mutagenicity tests using a multi-purpose strain of *Escherichia coli* K-12. *Mutat. Res.*, **19**, 257

132   MUTAGENESIS IN SUB-MAMMALIAN SYSTEMS

85. Fahrig, R. (1974). Development of host-mediated mutagenicity tests 1. Differential response of yeast cells injected into testes of rats and peritoneum of mice and rats to mutagens. *Mutat. Res.*, **25**, 29
86. Fahrig, R. (1977). Host-mediated mutagenicity tests – yeast systems. Recovery of yeast cells out of tests, liver, lung and peritoneum of rats. In: B. J. Kilbey, M. Legator, W. Nichols and C. Ramel (eds.). *Handbook of Mutagenicity Test Procedures*, pp. 135–147. (Amsterdam: Elsevier Biomedical Press, North-Holland)
87. Durston, W. and Ames, B. N. (1974). A simple method for detection of mutagens in urine, studies with the carcinogen 2-acetylamino-fluorine. *Proc. Natl. Acad. Sci. (USA)*, **71**, 737
88. Commoner, B., Vithayathil, A. J. and Henry, J. I. (1974). Detection of metabolic carcinogen intermediates in urine of carcinogen fed rats by means of bacterial mutagensis. *Nature (London)*, **249**, 850
89. Siebert, D. (1973). Induction of mitotic conversion in *Saccharomyces cerevisiae* by lymph fluid and urine of treated rats and human patients. *Mutat. Res.*, **21**, 202
90. Legator, M. S., Zimmering, S. and Connor, T. H. (1976). The use of indirect indicator systems to detect mutagenic activity in human subjects and experimental animals. In: A. Hollaender (ed.). *Chemical Mutagens, Principles and Methods for their Detection, Vol. 4*, pp. 174–191. (New York and London: Plenum Press)
91. Legator, M. S., Pullin, T. G. and Connor, T. H. (1977). The isolation and detection of mutagenic substances in body fluid and tissues of animals and body fluid of human subjects. In: B. J. Kilbey, M. Legator, W. Nichols and C. Ramel (eds.). *Handbook of Mutagenicity Test Procedures*, pp. 149–159. (Amsterdam: Elsevier Biomedical Press, North-Holland)
92. Bruce, W. R., Varghese, A. J., Furrer, R. and Land, P. C. (1977). A mutagen in the faeces of normal humans. In: H. H. Hiatt, J. D. Watson and J. A. Winsten (eds.). *Origins of Human Cancer, Vol. C*, pp. 1641–1646. (New York: Cold Spring Harbor Laboratory)
93. Evans, H. J. (1976). Cytological methods for detecting chemical mutagens. In: A. Hollaender (ed.). *Chemical Mutagens, Principles and Methods for their Detection, Vol. 4*, pp. 1–29. (New York and London: Plenum Press)
94. Bigani, M., Morpurgo, G., Pagliani, R., Carere, A., Conte, G. and Di Guiseppe, G. (1974). Non-disjunction and crossing-over induced by pharmaceutical drugs in *Aspergillis nidulans*. *Mutat. Res.*, **26**, 159
95. Parry, J. M. (1977). The detection of chromosome non-disjunction in the yeast *Saccharomyces cerevisiae*. In: D. Scott, B. A. Bridges and F. H. Sobels (eds.). *Progress in Genetic Toxicology*, pp. 223–229. (Amsterdam: Elsevier, Biomedical Press, North-Holland)
96. Parry, J. M. and Zimmerman, F. K. (1976). The detection of monosomic colonies produced by mitotic chromosome non-disjunction in the yeast *Saccharomyces cerevisiae*. *Mutat. Res.*, **35**, 49
97. Bond, D. J. (1976). System for the study of meiotic non-disjunction using *Sordaria brevicollis*. *Mutat. Res.*, **37**, 213
98. Kihlman, B. A. (1971). Root tips for studying the effects of chemicals on chromosomes. In: A. Hollaender (ed.). *Chemical Mutagens, Principles and*

TESTS OTHER THAN THE AMES TEST 133

Methods for their Detection, Vol. 2, pp. 489–514. (New York and London: Plenum Press)
99. Marimuthu, K. M., Sparrow, A. H. and Schairer, L. A. (1970). The cytological effects of space flight factors, vibration, clinostat and radiation on root tip cells of *Tradescantia*. *Radiation Res.*, **42**, 105
100. Ehrenberg, L. (1971). Higher plants. In: A. Hollaender (ed.). *Chemical Mutagens, Principles and Methods for their Detection, Vol. 2*, pp. 365–386. (New York and London: Plenum Press)
101. Nilan, R. A. and Vig, B. K. (1976). Plant test systems for detection of chemical mutagens. In: A. Hollaender (ed.). *Chemical Mutagens, Principles and Methods for their Detection, Vol. 4*, pp. 143–170. (New York and London: Plenum Press)
102. Würgler, F. E., Sobels, F. H. and Vogel, E. (1977). *Drosophila* as an assay system for detecting genetic changes. In B. J. Kilbey, M. Legator, W. Nichols and C. Ramel (eds.). *Handbook of Mutagenicity Test Procedures*. (Amsterdam: Elsevier Biomedical Press, North-Holland)
103. Smith, R. J. and Von Borstel, R. C. (1971). Inducing mutation with chemicals in *Habrobracon*. In: A. Hollaender (ed.). *Chemical Mutagens, Principles and Methods for their Detection, Vol. 2*, pp. 445–460. (New York and London: Plenum Press)
104. Von Borstel, R. C. and Smith, R. H. (1977). Measuring dominant lethality in *Habrobracon*. In B. J. Kilbey, M. Legator, W. Nichols and C. Ramel (eds.). *Handbook of Mutagenicity Testing Procedures*, pp. 375–387. (Amsterdam: Elsevier Biomedical Press, North-Holland)
105. Tazima, Y. and Onimaku, K. Results of mutagenicity testing for some nitrofuran derivatives in a sensitive test system with silkworm öocytes. *Japanese EMS 2nd Annual Meeting Abstract*, **14**, *Mutat. Res.*, **26** (1974) p. 440
106. Evans, H. J. and O'Riordan, M. L. (1975). Human peripheral blood lymphocytes for the analysis of chromosome aberrations in mutagen tests. *Mutat. Res.*, **31**, 135
107. Perry, P. and Evans, H. J. (1975). Cytological detection of mutagen–carcinogen exposure by sister chromatid exchange. *Nature (London)*, **258**, 121
108. Stetka, D. G. and Wolff, S. (1976). Sister chromatid exchange as an assay for genetic damage induced by mutagen–carcinogens. *Mutat. Res.*, **41**, 33
109. Cleaver, J. E. (1977). Methods for studying excision repair of DNA damaged by physical and chemical mutagens. In: B. J. Kilbey, M. Legator, W. Nichols and C. Ramel (eds.). *Handbook of Mutagenicity Test Procedures*, pp. 19–47. (Amsterdam: Elsevier Biomedical Press, North-Holland)
110. Cleaver, J. E. (1975) Methods for studying repair of DNA damaged by physical and chemical carcinogens. In: H. Busch (ed.). *Methods in Cancer Research, Vol. 9*, pp. 123–165. (New York: Academic Press)
111. Slater, E. Anderson, M. D. and Rosenkranz, H. S. (1971). Rapid detection of mutagens and carcinogens. *Cancer Res.*, **31**, 970
112. Kada, T., Morija, M. and Shirasu, Y. (1974). Screening of pesticides for DNA interactions by REC-assay and mutagenic testing and frameshift mutagens detected. *Mutat. Res.*, **26**, 243
113. Ichinotsubo, D., Mower, H. F., Setliff, J. and Mandel, M. (1977). The use of REC$^-$ bacteria for testing carcinogenic substances. *Mutat. Res.*, **46**, 53

114. Tanooka, J. (1977). Development and applications of *Bacillus subtilis* test system for mutagens involving DNA repair deficiency and suppressible auxotrophic mutations. *Mutat. Res.*, **48**, 367

115. Kafer, E., Marshall, P. and Cohen, G. (1976). Well marked strains of *Aspergillus* for tests of environmental mutagens: identification of induced recombination and mutation. *Mutat. Res.*, **38**, 141

116. Stich, H. F., San, R. H. C., Lam, P., Koropatnick, J. and Lo, L. (1977). Unscheduled DNA synthesis of human cells as a short-term assay for chemical carcinogens. In: H. H. Hiatt, J. D. Watson and J. A. Winsten (eds.). *Origins of Human Cancer, Vol. C*, pp. 1499–1512. (New York: Cold Spring Harbor Laboratory)

117. Purchase, I. F. H., Longstaff, E., Ashby, J., Styles, J. A., Anderson, D., Lefevre, P. A. and Westwood, F. R. (1978). An evaluation of six short-term tests for detecting organic chemical carcinogens. *Br. J. Cancer*, **37**, 873

118. Sugimura, T., Kawachi, T., Matsuskina, T., Nagao, M., Sate, S. and Yahagi, T. (1977). A critical review of sub-mammalian systems for mutagen detection. In: D. Scott, B. A. Bridges and F. H. Sobels (eds.). *Progress in Genetic Toxicology*, pp. 125–140. (Amsterdam: Elsevier Biomedical Press, North-Holland)

119. Russel, W. L. (1951). Specific locus mutations in mice. Cold Spring Harbor. *Quant. Biol.*, **16**, 327

120. Searle, A. G. (1975). The specific locus test in the mouse. *Mutat. Res.*, **31**, 277

121. Léonard, A. (1976). Test for heritable translocation in male mammals. *Mutat. Res.*, **31**, 291

122. Generso, W. M., Russell, W. L., Huff, S. W., Stout, S. R. and Gosslee, D. G. (1974). Effects of dose on the induction of dominant lethal mutations and heritable translocations with ethyl methanesulphonate in male mice. *Genetics*, **77**, 441

7

Cytogenetic aspects of mutagenicity testing
B. J. Dean

INTRODUCTION

Exposure of mammalian cells to mutagenic chemicals may result in a variety of detectable changes in the genetic material. The genetic changes to be described here are those involving whole chromosomes and are generally referred to as chromosome aberrations or anomalies. Unlike gene or point mutations, chromosome aberrations can be observed under a conventional light microscope at the metaphase stage of cell division (Figure 7.1).

At the metaphase stage of the cell cycle the chromosomes are discrete condensed objects in their most easily observable form. Each chromosome consists of an identical pair of chromatids joined by a single centromere. Chromosomes vary from each other in the length of the chromatids and in the position of the centromere along the chromosome, and these two parameters allow, in many cases, the identification of individual chromosomes.

Figure 7.2 shows the stages of cell division in an actively dividing mammalian cell.

This representation of the cell cycle shows that mitosis takes only a small proportion of the cycle. If, for example, the total period from one

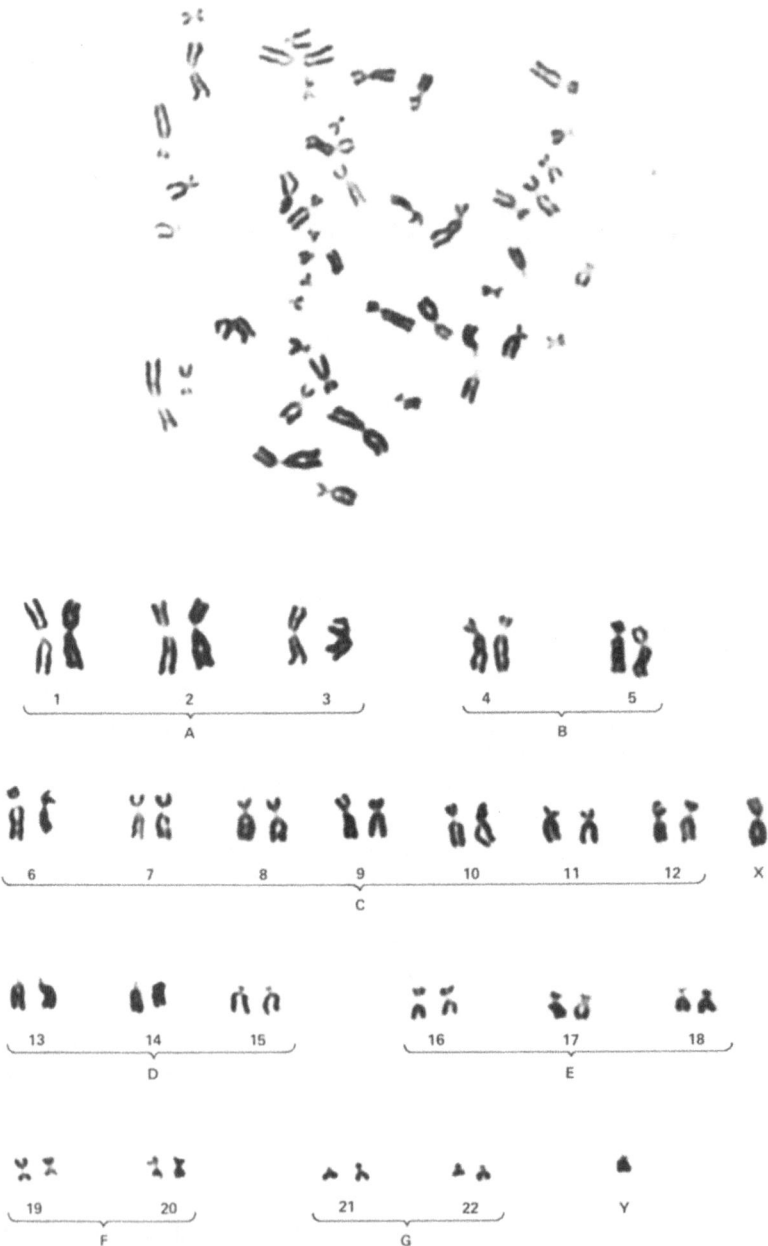

Figure 7.1 Human metaphase chromosomes (male)

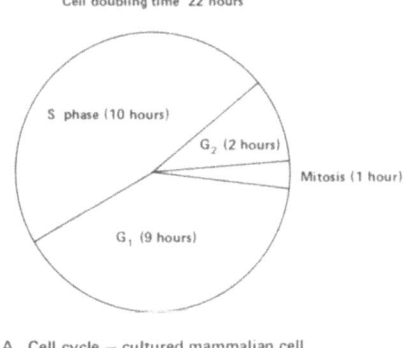

A. Cell cycle — cultured mammalian cell

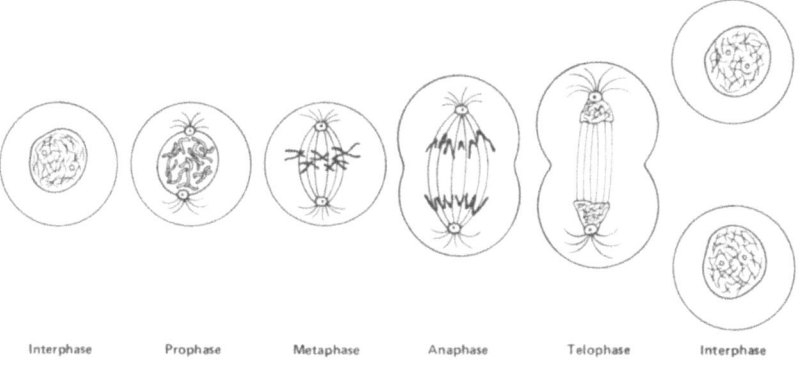

| Interphase | Prophase | Metaphase | Anaphase | Telophase | Interphase |

B. Mitotic cell division

Figure 7.2   Stages of cell division in a mammalian cell

division to the next is 22 h, the process of mitosis is complete in approximately 60 min and the metaphase chromosomes exist in an observable state for only a fraction of this. To obtain preparations suitable for microscopic analysis of metaphase chromosomes, i.e. with a high proportion of the cells at metaphase, it is necessary to use a metaphase-blocking agent such as colchicine, which leads to an accumulation of cells at this stage of mitosis as shown in Figure 7.3.

The technique of metaphase chromosome analysis, using colchicine or related chemicals, can be applied to rapidly dividing cells in laboratory animals and in cell cultures from mammals including man. It forms a basic procedure for detecting chemical-induced chromosome aberrations *in vivo* and, as will be described later, is used in conjunction with other short-term tests to provide a valuable *in vitro* assay for mutagenic chemicals.

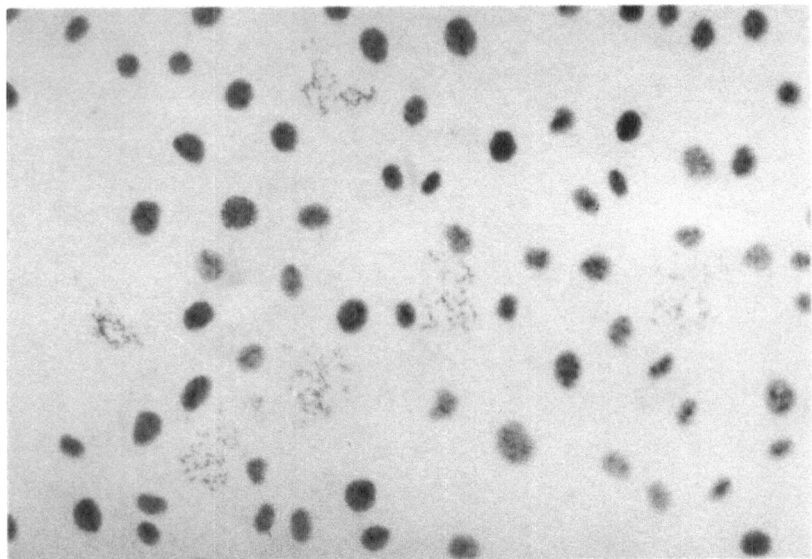

Figure 7.3   Metaphase accumulation in cell culture

CHROMOSOME ABERRATIONS

The chromosome anomalies with which we are concerned may be divided into either numerical or structural aberrations. Numerical aberrations are deviations from the normal diploid number for that species resulting in *aneuploidy* (random deviations) or *polyploidy* in which cells contain multiples of the haploid or diploid number of chromosomes.

Table 7.1 shows the chromosome number of species commonly used in chromosome studies ranging from a diploid number of 22 in the Chinese hamster to 78 in the dog.

Table 7.1   Chromosome numbers and polyploidy

	Haploid (n)	*Diploid* (2n)	*Tetraploid* (4n)
Chinese hamster	11	22	44
Mouse	20	40	80
Rat	21	42	84
Syrian hamster	22	44	88
Man	23	46	92
Dog	36	78	156

Polyploid $= 1n \times x$ Aneuploid $= 2n \pm x$

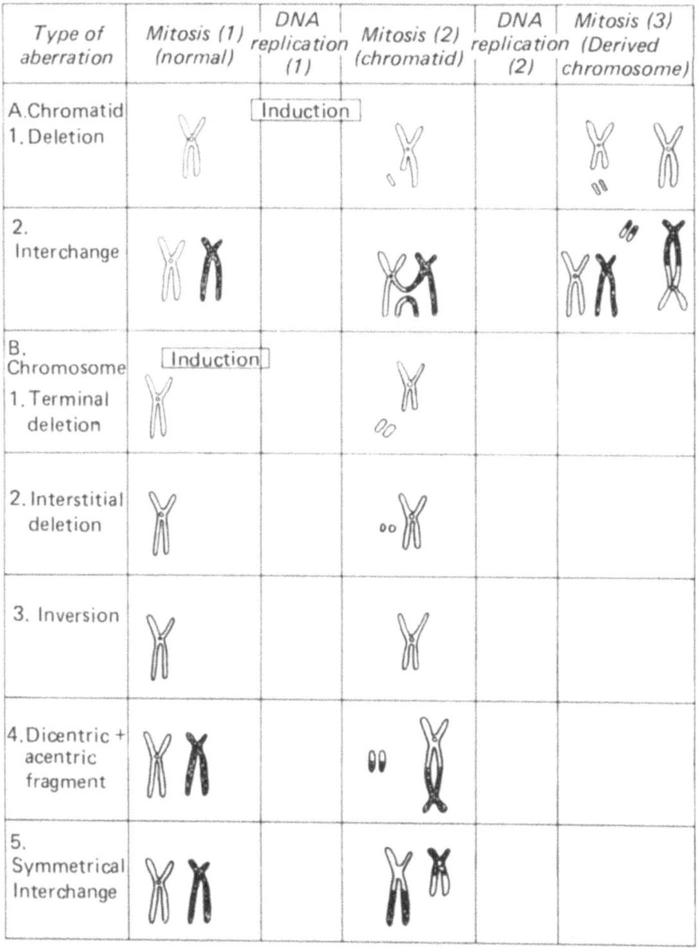

Type of aberration	Mitosis (1) (normal)	DNA replication (1)	Mitosis (2) (chromatid)	DNA replication (2)	Mitosis (3) (Derived chromosome)
A.Chromatid 1. Deletion		Induction			
2. Interchange					
B. Chromosome 1. Terminal deletion	Induction				
2. Interstitial deletion					
3. Inversion					
4. Dicentric + acentric fragment					
5. Symmetrical Interchange					

Figure 7.4 Structural chromosome and chromatid aberrations

Numerical anomalies result from errors occurring during cell division. If, for example, chromosome replication proceeds normally, yet the cell fails to divide, then the single 'daughter' cell will contain twice the diploid number of chromosomes (this is called *tetraploidy*, and in the more general case of a greater number of sets of chromosomes than four, polyploidy). Aneuploidy usually occurs as a result of inaccurate migration of chromosomes at anaphase so that one daughter cell will contain more and the other daughter cell fewer than the haploid or diploid number of chromosomes. Aneuploidy in human germ cells is responsible for a number of clinical syndromes which are discussed below.

Structural aberrations are caused primarily by chromosome breakage and rejoining of the broken chromosomes to form new configurations. Chromosome breakage can be induced by biological means (such as viruses), irradiation (such as ultraviolet, gamma-rays, X-rays) and by a wide variety of chemicals. The kinds of structural changes that are induced by exposure to mutagenic chemicals are influenced by the nature of the chemical, the stage in the cell cycle at which the damage is induced, and the number of cell divisions that occur between exposure to the chemical and observation of the damage.

Lesions induced by, for example, an alkylating agent during interphase (that is, the DNA synthesis S phase and G_2, Figure 7.2) appear at the next metaphase as chromatid aberrations, or aberrations of only one of the pair of chromatids that make up each chromosome. True chromosome aberrations are those that are observed at identical loci in each of the two chromatids and result from (a) damage induced before the DNA synthesis S phase and (b) replication of chromatid aberrations in the subsequent cell cycle. Examples of chromosome aberrations are shown in Figure 7.4.

CHROMOSOMES AND HUMAN DISEASE

It is necessary to stress that chromosomal anomalies play a significant role in the human disease burden. Almost all chromosome-related disease syndromes originate as chromosomal mutations in the parental germ cells

Table 7.2   Frequencies of chromosome anomalies in the newborn

Numerical changes	Chromosome complements	Frequency
Sex chromosome anomalies	XXY	1:400 (Klinefelter's syndrome)
	XXX	1:750
	XO	1:5000 (Turner's syndrome)
	XYY	1:2000
Autosomal trisomies	Trisomy 21	1:500 (Down's syndrome)
	Trisomy D13	1:8000 (Pateau's syndrome)
	Trisomy 18	1:5000 (Edward's syndrome)
Structural changes	Various structural aberrations with or without phenotypical changes	1:200 (e.g. deletion of short-arm of chromosome 5: (Cri-du-chat syndrome)

and the consequences range from early embryonic death to sex chromosome anomalies that may have no obvious ill-effects. In the most severe cases the progeny do not survive and if death occurs very early in embryonic development it may go completely unnoticed. Later in pregnancy, chromosome anomalies can be a direct cause of miscarriages, and estimates of the number of spontaneous abortions in which chromosome abnormalities have been identified vary from 30% to 50%[1]. Of the remainder one can only guess that a portion of them are due to mutations too small to detect by conventional metaphase analysis.

A small proportion of affected embryos survive to term often exhibiting one of a number of widely recognized clinical syndromes. Collectively these chromosomal mutations occur with an incidence of 0.5% of live births in the western world, and Table 7.2 illustrates some of them[2].

CHROMOSOMES AND CANCER

It has been known for many years that the cells of a number of types of neoplasms contain chromosomes that deviate structurally or numerically from the normal state. Polyploidy and aneuploidy are relatively common findings. In most cases the incidence and identity of the chromosome anomalies appear to be quite random and only rarely is a specific aberration common to a specific neoplasm. The best example of this is probably in chronic myeloid leukaemia in which the leukaemic cells contain a small group G chromosome, a segment of which has been transferred to another (usually a number 9) chromosome. This small, abnormal, group G chromosome is known as the Philadelphia chromosome[3].

It is important to emphasize that the Philadelphia chromosome occurs only in the leukaemic cells, and suggests very strongly the clonal origin of the disease.

It is also worth noting here that in many cases, individuals suffering from constitutional chromosome diseases are associated with a higher susceptibility to certain kinds of cancer than people in general. For example, individuals with Down's syndrome (mongolism) are estimated to have a twenty times greater risk of developing acute leukaemia[4] and males with Klinefelter's syndrome (or more than one X chromosome) exhibit a greater incidence of breast cancer than do normal males – though the incidence is very similar to that of normal females[5].

Many cases of familial retinoblastoma (a rare malignant tumour occurring in young children) occur in individuals who have a structural chromosome aberration in the form of a small deletion from a D-group chromosome[6].

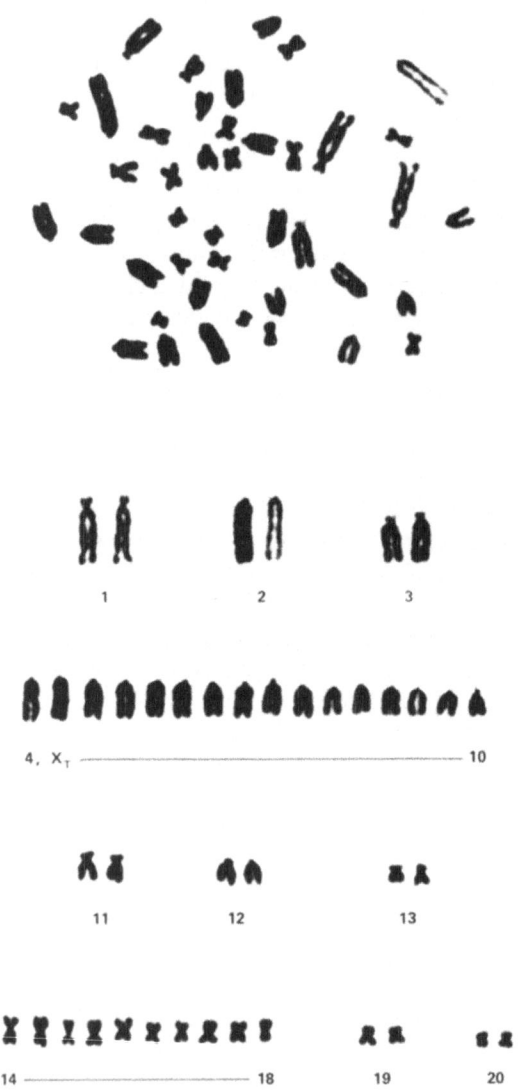

Figure 7.5   Metaphase chromosomes of the rat (female)

With the introduction of techniques that demonstrate the fine detail of chromosome structure, evidence has emerged of a relationship between chemical-induced chromosome lesions and the involvement of specific chromosome aberrations in neoplasia.

Specific regions of the largest telocentric rat chromosome are particularly sensitive to breakage by dimethylbenzanthracene (Figure 7.5). Dimethylbenzanthracene induces leukaemia and sarcomas in rats and the large telocentric chromosome is involved in both structural and numerical deviations in the malignant cells[7]. These facts strongly support the concept of a genetic mechanism in the development of the neoplasms but it is difficult at this stage to decide whether the chemical-induced chromosome lesions are directly responsible for the malignant changes by inducing an unbalanced genome or whether they are merely coincidental to more critical premalignant changes.

CHEMICAL-INDUCED CHROMOSOME DAMAGE

The role of chromosome anomalies in human disease has been discussed in some detail to illustrate the importance of assays of chromosome damage in any battery of short-term mutation assays. There is a tendency to disregard chromosome studies in favour of the more fashionable microbial mutation tests and cell transformation assays. One reason for this may be the concern that metaphase analysis is a time-consuming occupation which cannot be regarded as a rapid screening assay. On the contrary, *in vitro* chromosome assays using cultured mammalian cells are easily integrated into a screening system at a manpower cost comparable to that for a conventional microbial assay.

Examples of cultured cell systems that are well suited to screening chemicals are shown in Table 7.3.

Many chemicals require some degree of metabolic alteration before an

Table 7.3   *In vitro* **chromosome assays**

Source of cells	Cell type	Metabolic activation*
Human	Lymphocyte	Absent or add S-9
Chinese hamster	Fibroblasts	Absent or add S-9
Mouse	Fibroblasts	Absent or add S-9
Syrian hamster embryo	Mixed types	Intrinsic
Rat liver (RL$_1$)	Epithelial	Intrinsic

* S-9 = Microsomal enzyme fraction of rat liver homogenate

active molecule is generated and this may be introduced into the test-system in the form of microsomal enzymes derived from rat liver or by using cells which are metabolically competent. The latter method has the advantage that both the metabolic activation and the genetic change can take place in the same cell. A method developed at Tunstall Laboratory and used routinely for almost 3 years, utilizes a cell line derived from rat liver. The cells contain residual metabolizing enzyme activity and, as can be seen from Table 7.4, are sensitive to chromosome breakage by a variety of chemical mutagens and carcinogens.

Table 7.4   Chemical-induced chromatid aberrations in rat liver (RL₁) cells

Compound	Dose (μg/m)l	Percentage of cells with chromatid deletions and interchanges	Microbial mutation −S-9 +S-9	
Control	—	0–0.3	—	—
Methyl methanesulphonate	10	20.0	+	+
Methyl nitronitosoguanine	1	6.5	+	+
4-Nitroquinoline-N-oxide	0.04	5.2	+	+
2-Acetylaminofluorene	30	10.5	−	+
3-Methylcholanthrene	4	3.1	−	+
7,12-Dimethylbenz(a)anthracene	12.5	5.5	−	+
Cyclophosphamide	2000	10.3	−	+
Pyrene	100	0	−	−
Carbon tetrachloride	0.02	0	−	−

It must be emphasized that there are a number of chemicals, such as benzene and urethane, that are known to induce chromosome aberrations in mammals – including man – and which fail to produce a positive response in microbial mutation tests.

CONCLUSION

In this paper I have discussed mammalian chromosomes and the morphological changes that can be induced in chromosomes in biological, physical and chemical agents. I have described very briefly some of the consequences of chromosome anomalies for man and reviewed some simple *in vitro* tests by which chemicals can be screened for their ability to damage mammalian chromosomes. I hope I have succeeded in illustrating the importance of including tests for chemical-induced chromosome damage in any battery of tests designed to screen chemicals for possible mutagenic or carcinogenic hazard.

References

1. Carr, D. H. (1970). Chromosome abnormalities and spontaneous abortions. In: P. A. Jacobs, W. H. Price and P. Law (eds.). *Human Population Cytogenetics*, pp. 103–118. (Edinburgh: University Press)
2. Vogel, F. (1970). Spontaneous mutations in man. In: F. Vogel and G. Röhrborn (eds.). *Chemical Mutagenesis in Man and Mammals*, pp. 16–68. (Berlin, Heidelberg, New York: Springer-Verlag)
3. Nowell, P. C. and Hungerford, D. A. (1970). A minute chromosome in human chronic granulocytic leukaemia. *Science, NY*, **132**, 1497
4. Holland, W. W., Doll, R. and Carter, C. O. (1962). The mortality from leukaemia and other cancers among patients with Down's syndrome (mongols) and among their parents. *Br. J. Cancer*, **16**, 177
5. Lynch, H. T., Kaplan, A. R. and Lynch, J. F. (1974). Klinefelter's syndrome and cancer. A family study. *J. Am. Med. Assoc.*, **229**, 809
6. Atkin, N. B. (1976). *Cytogenetic Aspects of Malignant Transformation*, pp. 23. (Basel: S. Karger)
7. Sugiyama, T. (1971). Specific vulnerability of the largest telocentric chromosome of rat bone marrow cells to 7,12-dimethyl-benz(a)anthracene. *J. Natl. Cancer Inst.*, **47**, 1267

Recommended reading

Bartalos, M. and Baramki, T. A. (1967). *Medical Cytogenetics*. (Baltimore: Williams and Wilkins Company)
Evans, H. J. and O'Riordan, M. L. (1977). Human peripheral blood lymphocytes for the analysis of chromosome aberrations in mutagen tests. In: B. J. Kilbey, M. Legator, W. Nichols, and C. Ramel (eds.). *Handbook of Mutagenicity Test Procedures*, pp. 261–274. (Amsterdam, New York, Oxford: Elsevier)
Evans, H. J. (1976). Cytological methods for detecting chemical mutagens. In: A. Hollaender (ed.). *Chemical Mutagens, Principles and Methods for their Detection, Vol. 4*, pp. 1–29. (New York and London: Plenum Press)
Jacobs, P. A., Price, W. H. and Law, P. (eds.). (1970). *Human Population Cytogenetics*. (Edinburgh: University Press)
Yunis, J. J. (1977). *Molecular Structure of Human Chromosomes*. (New York, San Francisco, London: Academic Press)
Yunis, J. J. (ed.) (1974). *Human Chromosome Methodology*, 2nd ed. (New York and London: Academic Press)

8

Cell transformation assays
J. A. Styles

INTRODUCTION

A number of cell culture systems have been developed over the past ten years in which normal or non-malignant cells have been changed ('transformed') with respect to various test markers, including malignancy in the whole animal, following injection of the cells after exposure *in vitro* to chemical carcinogens. The prime purpose of these methods was the analysis of the mechanisms involved in chemical carcinogenesis but they also showed great promise as rapid tests to detect potential carcinogens.

The early investigations into the phenomenon of cell transformation were concerned with observing changes in morphology of the test cells and alterations in the growth patterns of the colonies formed following exposure to carcinogens. Two morphological transformation systems have been studied extensively; the first, using, Syrian hamster embryonic cells, has been reviewed by Di Paolo[1,2] and the second, using mouse cells (C3H/10T$\frac{1}{2}$) has been reviewed by Heidelberger[3-5]. Many carcinogens have been correctly identified using this type of assay as a screen[6].

Later developments in test methodology introduced other endpoints and some of these are listed in Table 8.1. Most of the data on the various indicators of transformation are based on embryonic fibroblast cells although more recent work on these endpoints has concentrated on epithelial cells, since it has been estimated that 85% of human cancers are

Table 8.1   Properties of transformed cells in culture

Cell properties	Fibroblasts	Epithelial cells	Correlation with tumorigenicity
Tumorigenicity	+	+	
Growth in agar or methocel	+	+	.98
Morphological changes	+	−	<.75
Increased saturation density and piling-up	+	±	<.75
Decreased serum requirement	+	?	<.75
Altered cell-surface glycoproteins and glycolipids	+	?	?
Lectin agglutination	+	+	?
Increased membrane transport	+	?	?
Decreased cAMP	+	?	?
Increased protease production	+	?	<.75
Decreased microfilament sheaths	+	?	?

epithelial in origin[7,8]. The relevance of any *in vitro* transformation end-point to cancer can be tested by taking the cells, implanting them into suitable animal hosts and observing the appearance of tumours. Growth in semi-solid agar appears, at the moment, to be the most reliable criterion for transformation of both fibroblast and epithelial cultures and has the best correlation with tumorigenicity (0.98), whereas the other test end-points had correlation coefficients of less than 0.75[9,10]. Growth in agar is a simple and objective criterion of transformation but does not detect early changes in cells following exposure to a chemical carcinogen[11,12]. The different markers of neoplastic transformation listed in Table 8.1 are acquired by primary or early passage cells after various population doublings following exposure to a carcinogen but the last characteristic to appear is the ability to grow in semi-solid agar[10]. It is assumed that the lesion caused by the carcinogen in primary or early passage cells is followed by a series of independent steps leading to malignant transformation. If established cell lines such as BHK21 Cl 13 or CHO-K1 cells are exposed to a carcinogen then transformation occurs rapidly, indicating that these cells are very near to the transformed state (Figure 8.1). This is borne out by the observation that BHK cells have a relatively high spontaneous transformation frequency and can produce tumours in hamsters if large numbers of cells are inoculated, whereas primary cells show little or no spontaneous transformation and are not tumorigenic.

Of the available short-term predictive tests for carcinogens which have been validated[6,13−22], cell transformation assays have an obvious demonstrable connection with cancer, which may be useful when relating the

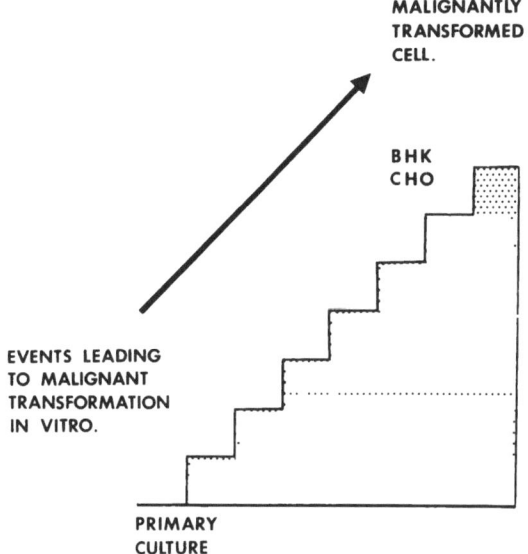

MALIGNANTLY
TRANSFORMED
CELL.

BHK
CHO

EVENTS LEADING
TO MALIGNANT
TRANSFORMATION
IN VITRO.

PRIMARY
CULTURE

INCREASING NUMBER OF CELL GENERATIONS

Figure 8.1 Schematic diagram of malignant transformation *in vitro*. The events leading to transformation, some of which are listed in Table 8.1, are known to occur after a single exposure to a carcinogen. The last event is thought to be growth in semi-solid agar

in vitro positive test result of a compound to the induction of a tumour. However desirable it may be to have a short-term test which is related to cancer, for the purposes of a screen the main concern should be initially an ability to discriminate between carcinogens and non-carcinogens.

A clear distinction must be drawn, for the present, between *in vitro* cell transformation studies which are directed towards understanding the mechanisms of carcinogenesis and those which are used to detect chemical carcinogens, particularly when established cell lines are used. These cells are metabolically abnormal and may be used in conjunction with liver homogenates (S 9 mix) to augment metabolism, in which case the magnitude of the test response will be determined largely by the balance between activating and detoxifying enzymes in the S 9 mix. It must also be borne in mind that any cell culture model is a simplified version of the intact animal and while models may be useful as a means of solving specific problems in toxicology, the results derived from *in vitro* studies must not be extrapolated beyond the limits of the system. The cell culture transformation models described above are closed systems and are lacking in most of the barriers that a chemical must pass through in an animal before reaching the target macromolecules critical to cancer induction (route of entry, absorption, 'real' metabolism, detoxification and excretion) and the barriers that a population of exposed cells must negotiate before a malignant tumour appears (cellular repair, immunosurveillance, humoral controls).

BHK CELL TRANSFORMATION ASSAY

The BHK transformation system, using growth in semi-solid agar as an endpoint will serve as an example of how cell transformation assays can be used to screen chemicals for carcinogenic potential and to gather experimental evidence for structure-activity studies. The BHK-agar transformation assay[23-25] has been modified to include auxiliary metabolic activation[22], and has been subjected to a validation study using 120 chemicals[20,21] where it was found to be capable of discriminating between carcinogens and non-carcinogens with about 90% accuracy. Similar accuracy has been reported by Pienta[6] using Syrian hamster embryo cells and observing morphological transformation. Figures indicating predictive accuracy in short-term tests must be treated with

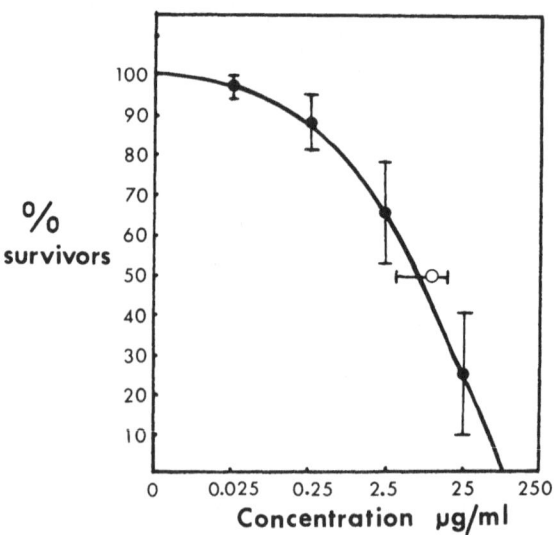

Figure 8.2 Survival curve of BHK cells exposed to benzo(a)pyrene for 3 h. Mean of ten experiments ± SD

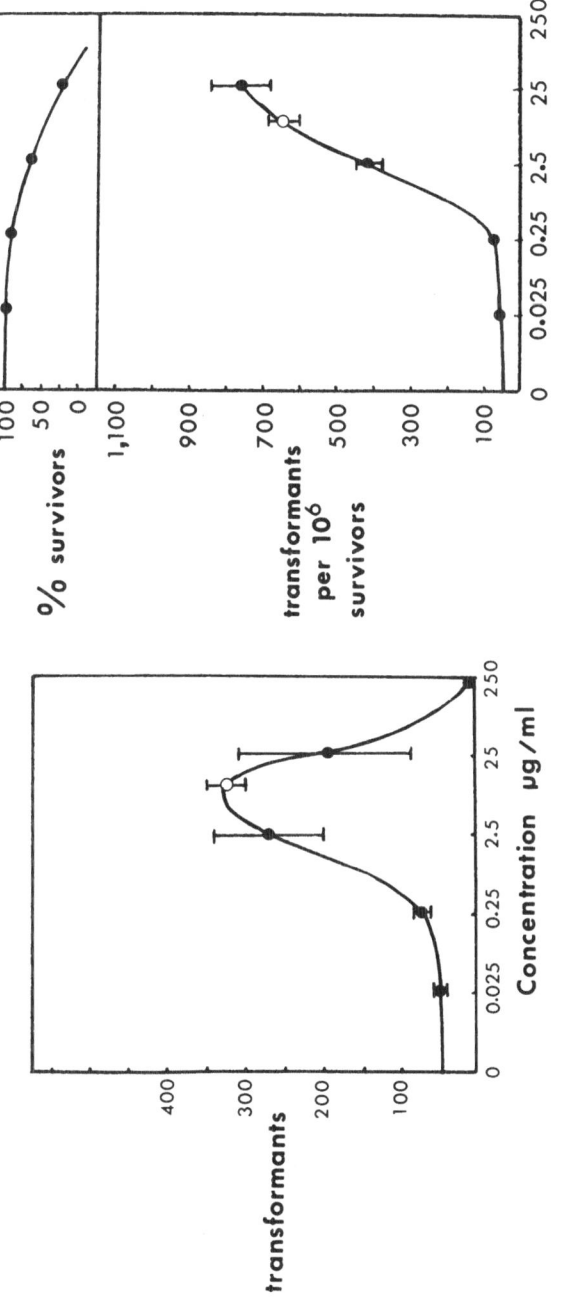

Figure 8.4 Transformation frequency of BHK cells after treatment with benzo(a)pyrene. Mean of ten experiments ± SD

Figure 8.3 Number of colonies of BHK cells growing in semi-solid agar after treatment with benzo(a)pyrene. Mean of ten experiments ± SD

caution since they can be altered by the choice of chemicals used[26]. It has been proposed[21,27] that maximum reliance can be placed on the prediction from a short-term test only if carcinogenic and non-carcinogenic structural analogues of the test chemical are assayed at the same time and give the correct response. Obviously, if the control analogues behave incorrectly in the assay, little reliance can be placed on the result generated by the test compound.

The reliability of the cell transformation test using BHK cells can be seen from Figures 8.2 to 8.4. The results of testing benzo(a)pyrene on ten separate occasions are shown in these figures. It can be seen from the survival curve in Figure 8.2 that the accuracy declines at low survival but that it is possible to determine the LC_{50} within a 10-fold dose range. All test results are compared at the LC_{50} so that differences in toxicity between compounds are eliminated. Figure 8.3 shows the number of transformed colonies found in semi-solid agar following incubation of BHK cells with benzo(a)pyrene. The transformation frequency derived from the previous

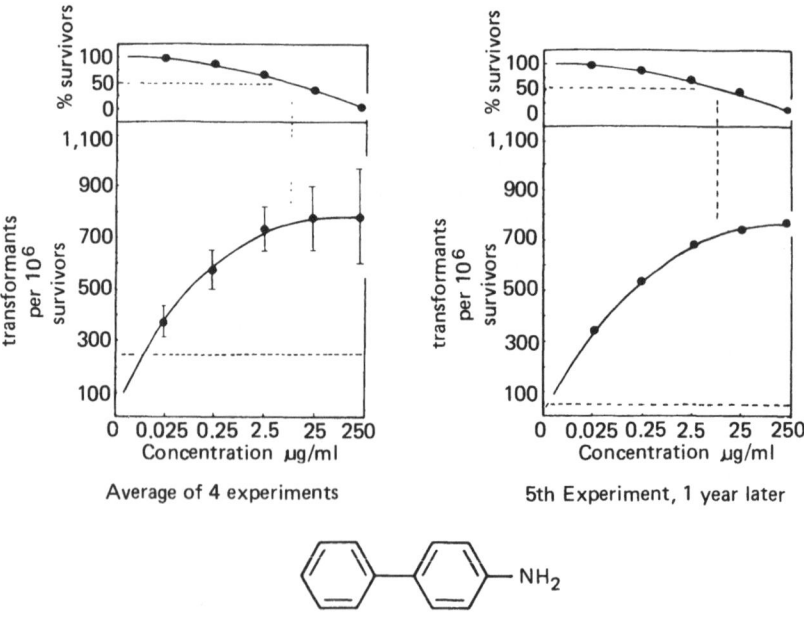

Figure 8.5 Comparison of transformation assays on 4-aminobiphenyl with a clone of BHK cells which had a spontaneous transformation frequency of 50 per 10^6 cells and with a clone having a spontaneous transformation frequency of 10 per 10^6 cells

two sets of data is shown in Figure 8.4, where it can be seen that transformation and survival are interdependent since the errors at all doses are greatly reduced. Similar results have also been obtained with 2-acetylaminofluorene and benzidine.

Since BHK cells transform spontaneously, a population of BHK cells maintained continuously in culture will accumulate transformants, so recloning and selection must be carried out regularly[28,29]. Recloning does not appear to affect the sensitivity of the cells as can be seen in Figure 8.5 where the results of testing 4-aminobiphenyl in a clone of cells having a spontaneous transformation frequency of 50 per 10^6 cells (that is, a threshold frequency of 250 per 10^6 survivors at the LC_{50}[22] are compared with the results of a test carried out about a year later on 4-aminobiphenyl, using a clone of cells with a spontaneous transformation frequency of 10 per 10^6 cells (that is, a threshold frequency of 50 per 10^6 survivors at the LC_{50}). These results also demonstrate the reproducibility of the test.

COMPARISON WITH BACTERIAL ASSAY

There are many classes of chemical carcinogens which are correctly distinguished by both the cell transformation assay and the *Salmonella* test (83% of compounds tested by Purchase *et al.*[21]) examples being tobacco smoke condensate (Figure 8.6), *para*-nitrosodimethylaniline (Figure 8.7), vinyl chloride (Figure 8.8), unstabilized trichlorethylene (Figure 8.9), ethylene dichloride (Figure 8.10), and chloroform (Figure 8.11). However, when compared with the *Salmonella* assay it can be seen that for certain classes of chemicals the cell transformation assay can discriminate between carcinogens and non-carcinogens which are not detected by the bacterial assay. For example, the cell transformation assay distinguished between the non-carcinogen aniline and the closely related carcinogen *o*-toluidine. The response of this test for an untested aniline is therefore credible, in contrast to the *Salmonella* assay which registers both aniline and *o*-toluidine as negative or positive depending on the test conditions or whether or not norharman is included[30-32]. In both situations the result from the *Salmonella* assay for a previously untested aniline is of indeterminate significance (Figures 8.12 and 8.13). A further example of a carcinogen which the cell transformation assay is capable of detecting correctly, but which gave negative results in the *Salmonella* assay, was 2-aminotriazole. Based on this test response it is possible to predict that a structurally related, but untested analogue of 2-aminotriazole, guanazole will be non-carcinogenic (Figures 8.14 and 8.15).

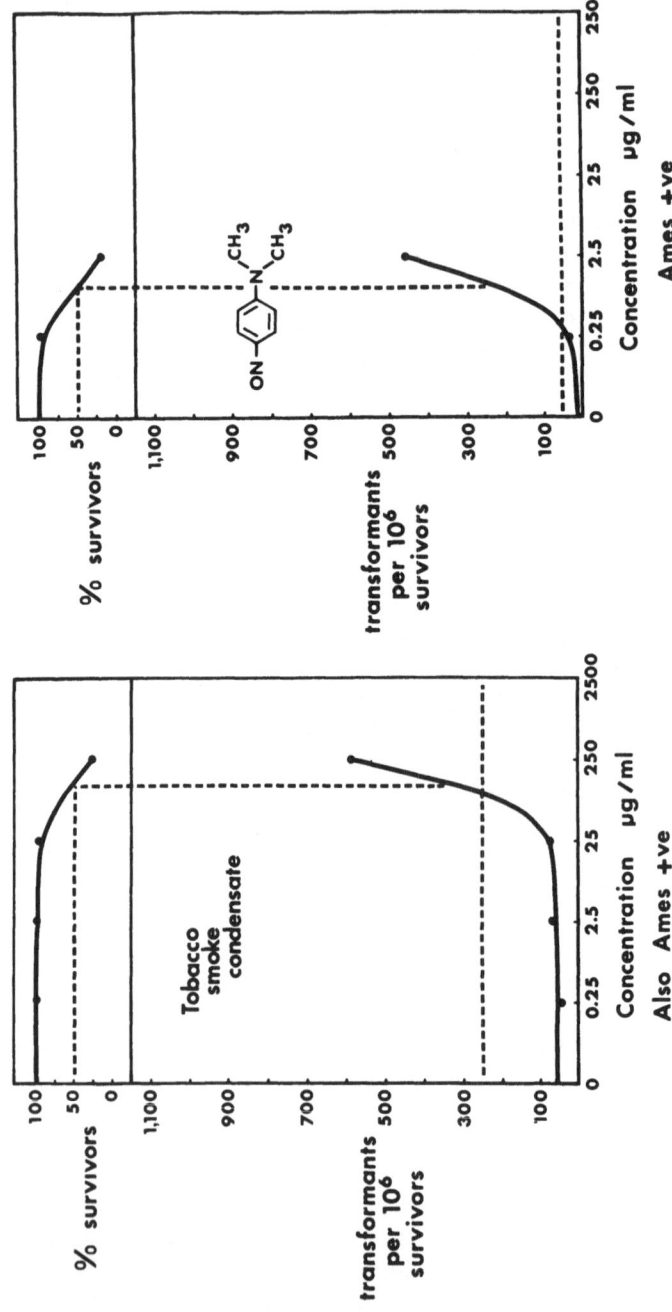

Figure 8.6 Transformation assay of tobacco smoke condensate. A positive result was also found in the Ames' assay

Figure 8.7 Transformation assay of *para*nitrosodimethylaniline showing positive result. The Ames' assay was also positive

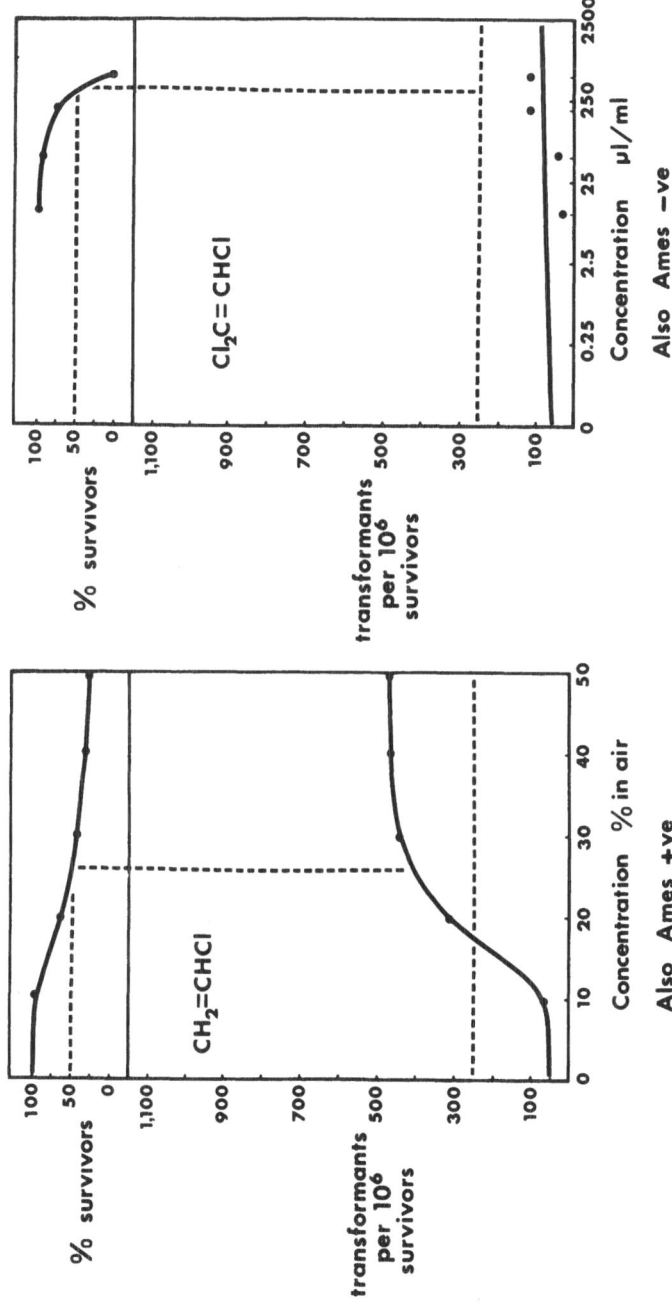

Figure 8.8 Transformation assay of vinyl chloride gas. Both the transformation and Ames' assays gave positive results

Figure 8.9 Negative result given by unstabilized trichlorethylene in transformation assay. Unstabilized TCE also gave a negative result in Ames' assay

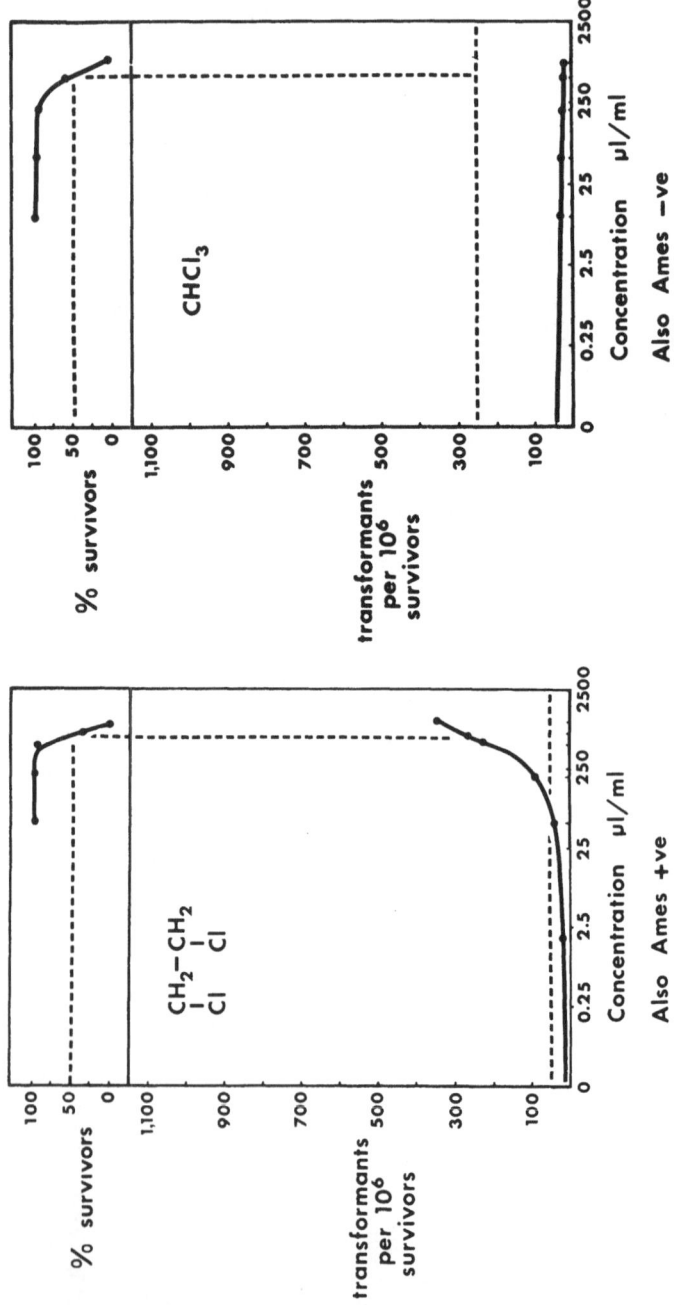

Figure 8.10 Positive transformation result with ethylene di-chloride which was also positive in the Ames' assay

Figure 8.11 Negative result in transformation assay of chloroform which was also negative in the Ames' assay

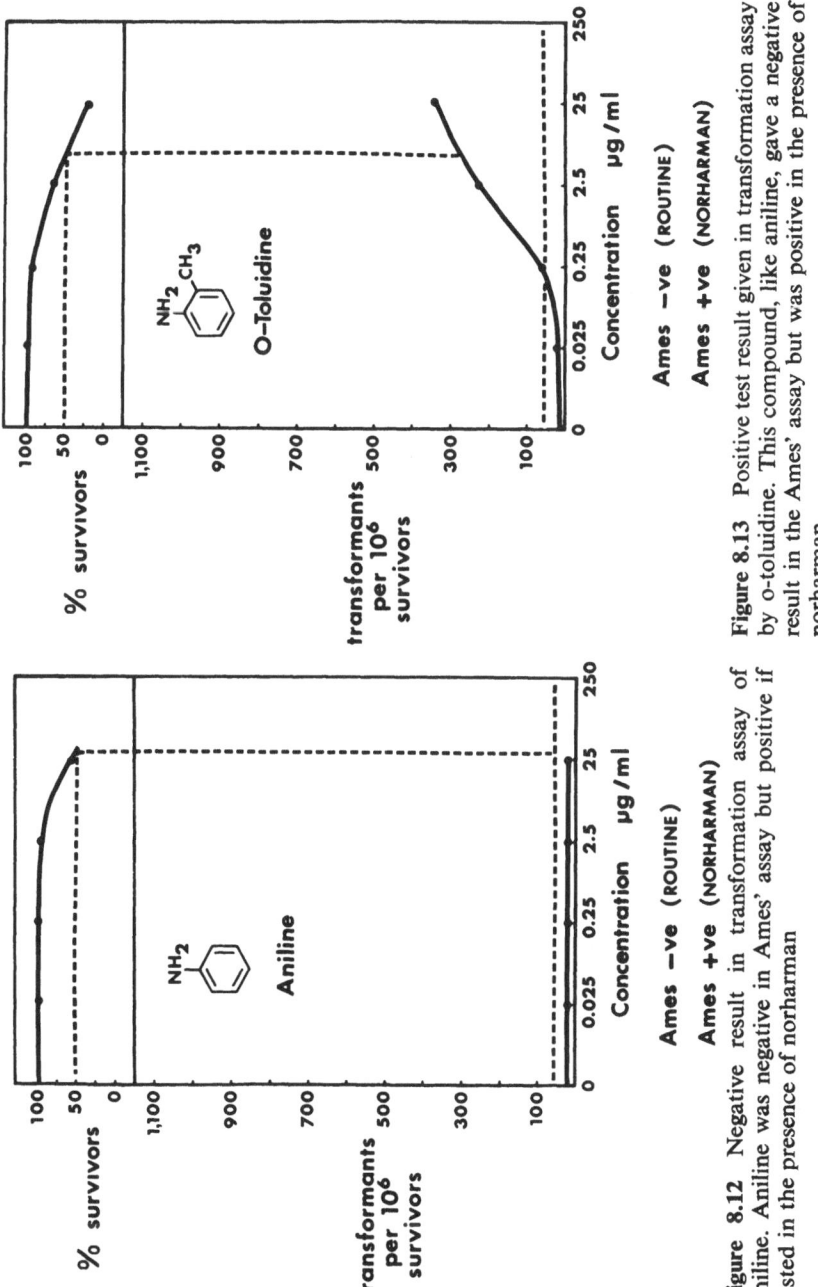

Figure 8.12 Negative result in transformation assay of aniline. Aniline was negative in Ames' assay but positive if tested in the presence of norharman

Figure 8.13 Positive test result given in transformation assay by o-toluidine. This compound, like aniline, gave a negative result in the Ames' assay but was positive in the presence of norharman

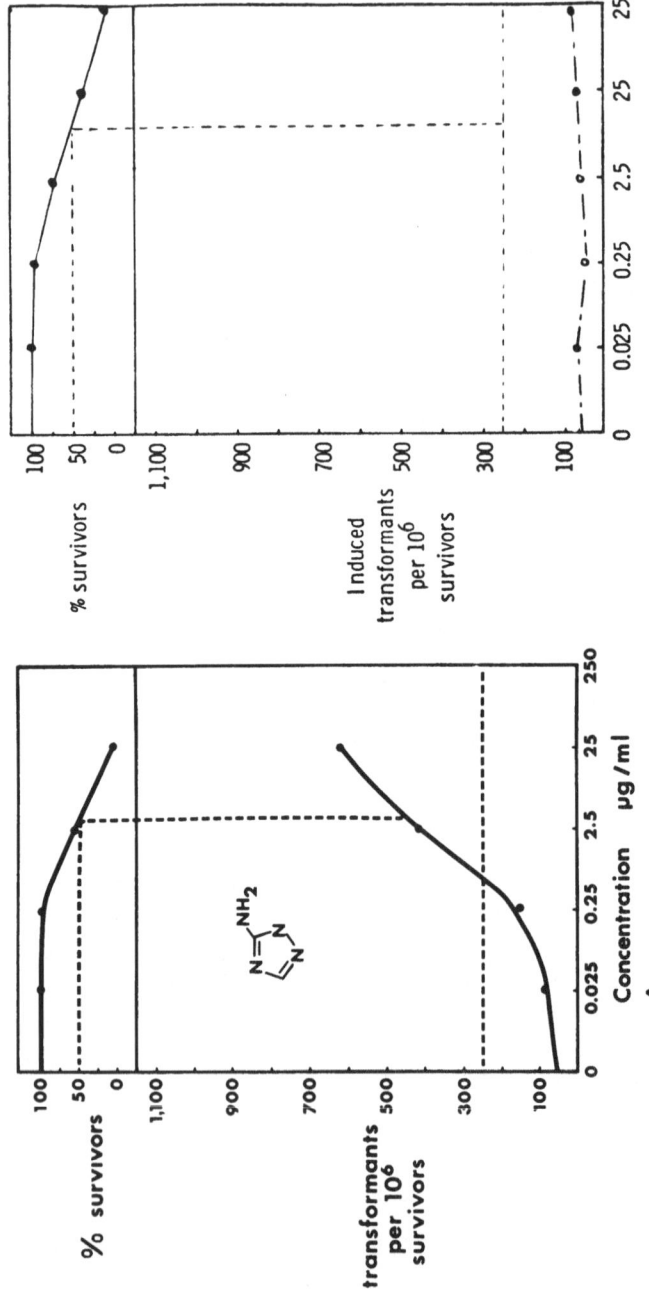

Figure 8.14 Positive transformation assay result given by 2-aminotriazole which is Ames' negative

Figure 8.15 Negative transformation assay result given by guanazole, a non-carcinogenic analogue of 2-aminotriazole. Guanazole was also negative in the Ames' assay

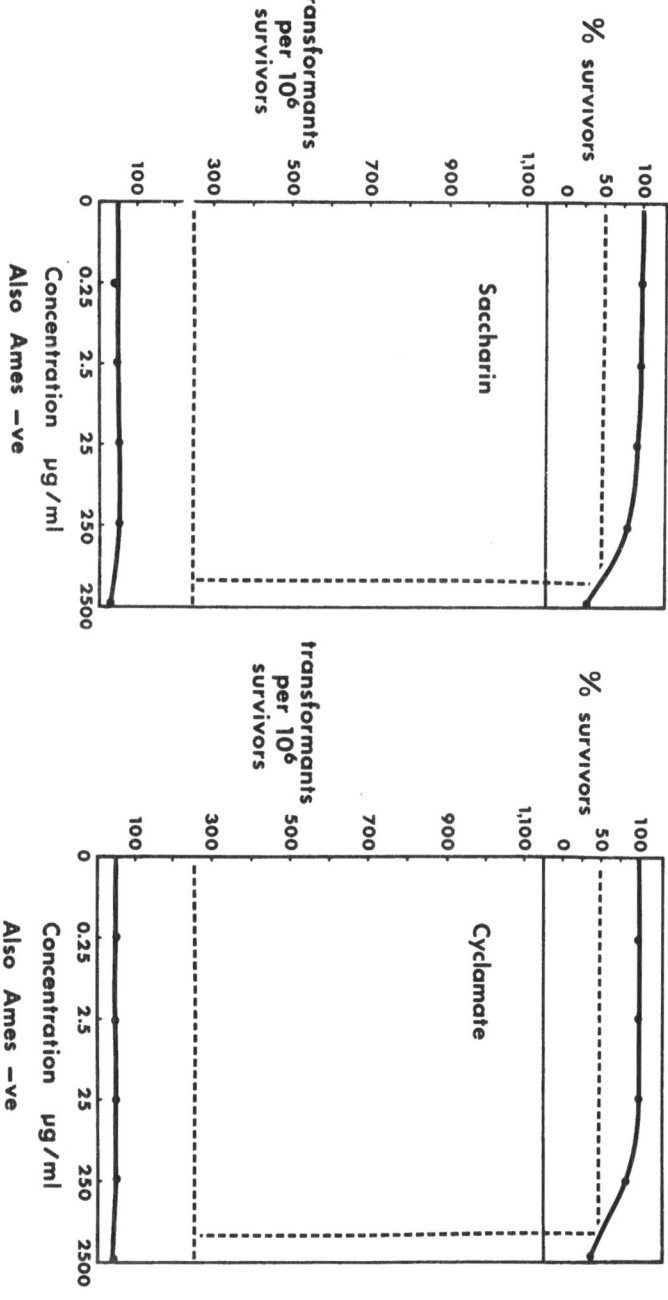

Figure 8.16 Negative test results given in cell transformation assay and Ames' test with saccharin

Figure 8.17 Negative test result given in cell transformation assay and Ames' test with cyclamate

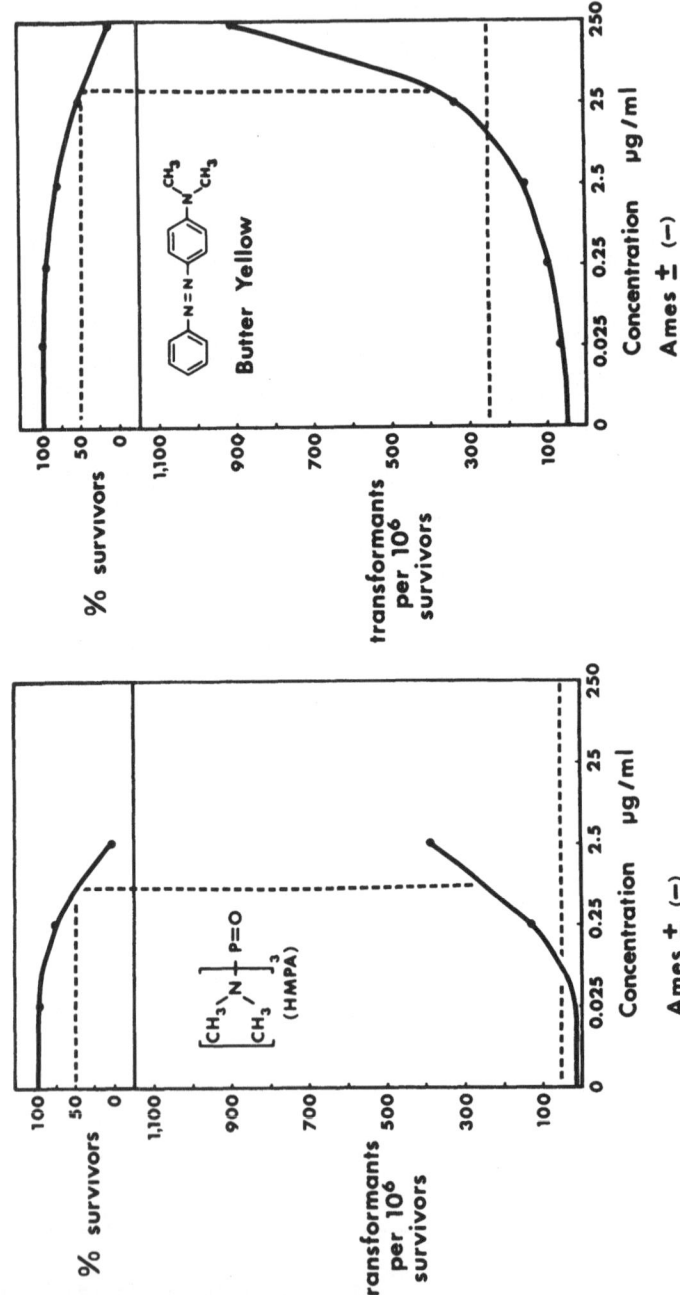

Figure 8.18 The carcinogen hexamethyl phosphoramide (HMPA) is consistently positive in the cell transformation assay but is erratic and mainly negative in the Ames' test

Figure 8.19 The carcinogen butter yellow gives a consistently positive result in the cell transformation assay but is erratic and mainly negative in the Ames' test

There are compounds such as saccharin and cyclamate which have produced tumours in animals but which are negative in both the *Salmonella* and cell transformation assays (Figures 8.16 and 8.17). It has been argued that these compounds are epigenetic carcinogens and would not be expected to register in short-term tests such as those above which are probably sensitive to genotypic carcinogens[33].

Further categories of chemical carcinogens give reproducible positive results in the cell transformation assay whilst giving erratic but mainly negative results in the *Salmonella* test, examples being hexamethylphosphoramide (Figure 8.18), butter yellow (Figure 8.19), dimethylnitrosamine and hydrazine. However, it must be noted that the cell transformation assay failed to detect some other classes of carcinogen, such as the flame retardant *tris* (2,3-dibromopropyl) phosphate and trimethyl phosphate which are correctly identified by the *Salmonella* assay.

In summary, the BHK cell transformation test, as an example of mammalian cell transformation assays, is reproducible and gives good discrimination between carcinogens and non-carcinogens of many classes. The assay should be used, where possible, with appropriate chemical class controls (as should any short-term test) in order to increase the credibility of the test result for a compound of undefined activity.

Finally, since the cell transformation test is a simpler system than the whole animal and does not employ the full metabolic capacity of an intact mammal, the magnitude of the test response is of unknown relevance and should not be assumed, in the present state of knowledge, to define the potency of a carcinogen.

References

1. Di Paolo, J. A. (1974a). Quantitative aspects of *in vitro* chemical carcinogenesis. *Biochem. Dis.*, **4**, 443
2. Di Paolo, J. A. (1974b). Quantitative aspects of *in vitro* chemical carcinogenesis. In: P.O.P. Ts'o and J. A. Di Paolo (eds.). *Chemical Carcinogenesis (Part B)* pp. 443–455. (New York: Marcel Dekker Inc.)
3. Heidelberger, C. (1973a). Chemical oncogenesis in culture. *Adv. Cancer Res.*, **18**, 317
4. Heidelberger, C. (1973b). Current trends in chemical carcinogenesis; *Fed. Proc.* **32**, 2154
5. Heidelberger, C. (1975). Chemical carcinogenesis. *Ann. Rev. Biochem.*, **44**, 79
6. Pienta (personal communication)
7. Cairns, J. (1975). The cancer problem. *Sci. Am.*, **233**, 64
8. Higginson, J. and Muir, C. S. (1973). Epidermology. In: J. F. Holland and E. Frei, III (eds.), *Cancer Medicine*, p. 241. (Philadelphia: Lea and Febiger)

9. Ts'o, P.O.P. (1977). Some aspects of the basic mechanisms of chemical carcinogenesis. *J. Toxicol. Env. Hlth*, **2**, 1305
10. Ts'o, P.O.P. (1978). The relationship between neoplastic transformation and the cellular genetic apparatus. Paper given at the American Tissue Culture Association 29th Annual meeting, 1978
11. Weinstein, I. B., Wigler, M. and Stadler, U. (1976). Analysis of the mechanism of chemical carcinogenesis in epithelial cell cultures. In: R. Montesano, H. Bartsch, and L. Tomatis. *Screening Tests in Chemical Carcinogenesis.* IARC/WHO Scientific Publication No. 12
12. Weinstein, B., Yamaguchi, N., Gebert, R. and Kaighn, M. E. (1975). Use of epithelial cell cultures for studies on the mechanism of transformation by chemical carcinogens. *In vitro*, **11**, 130
13. Brookes, P. and de Serres, F. (1976). Report on the workshop on the mutagenicity of chemical carcinogens, Honolulu 1974. *Mutation Res.*, **88**, 155
14. Stoltz, D. R., Poirier, L. A., Irving, C. C., Stich, H. F., Weisburger, J. H. and Grice, H. C. (1974). Evaluation of short-term tests for carcinogenicity. *Toxicol. Appl. Pharmacol.*, **29**, 157
15. Montesano, R., Bartsch, H. and Tomatis, L. (1976). *Screening Tests in Chemical Carcinogenesis.* IARC/WHO Scientific Publication No. 12
16. Ames, B. N., Durston, W. E., Yamasaki, E. and Lee, F. D. (1973). Carcinogens are mutagens: A simple test system combining liver homogenates for activation and bacteria for detection. *Proc. Natl. Acad. Sci. (USA)*, **70**, 228
17. Ames, B. N., McCann, J. and Yamasaki, E. (1975). Methods for detecting carcinogens and mutagens with the *Salmonella*/mammalian–microsome mutagenicity test. *Mutation Res.*, **31**, 347
18. McCann, J., Choi, E., Yamasaki, E. and Ames, B. N. (1975). Detection of carcinogens as mutagens in the *Salmonella*/microsome test Part 1, assay of 300 chemicals. *Proc. Natl. Acad. Sci. (USA)*, **72**, 5135
19. McCann, J. and Ames, B. N. (1976). Detection of carcinogens as mutagens in the *Salmonella*/microsome test: Assay of 300 chemicals: Part II discussion. *Proc. Natl. Acad. Sci. (USA)*, **73**, 950
20. Purchase, I. F. H., Longstaff, E., Ashby, J., Styles, J. A., Anderson, D., Lefevre, P. A., and Westwood, F. E. (1976). Evaluation of six short-term tests for detecting organic chemical carcinogens and recommendations for their use. *Nature (London)*, **264**, 624
21. Purchase, I. F. H., Longstaff, E. Ashby, J., Styles, J. A., Anderson, D., Lefevre, P. A. and Westwood, F. R. (1978). Evaluation of six short-term tests for detecting organic chemical carcinogens and recommendations for their use. *Br. J. Cancer*, **37**, 873
22. Styles, J. A. (1977). A method for detecting carcinogenic organic chemicals using mammalian cells in culture. *Br. J. Cancer*, **36**, 558
23. Macpherson, I. and Montagnier, L. (1964). Agar suspension culture for the selective assay of cells transformed by polyoma virus. *Virology*, **23**, 291
24. Di Mayorca, G., Greenblatt, M., Trauthen, T., Soller, A. and Giordano, R. (1973). Malignant transformation of BHK 21 Clone 13 cells *in vitro* by nitrosamines – a conditional state. *Proc. Natl. Acad. Sci. (USA)*, **70**, 46
25. Mishra, N. K. and Di Mayorca, G. (1974). *In vitro* malignant transformation of cells by chemical carcinogens. *Biochem. Biophys. Acta*, **355**, 205
26. Ashby, J. (1978). (Chapter 9, this volume)

27. Ashby, J. and Purchase, I. F. H. (1977). The selection of appropriate chemical class controls for use with short-term tests for potential carcinogenicity. *Ann. Occup. Hygiene*, **20**, 297
28. Bouck, N. and Di Mayorca, G. (1976). Somatic mutation as the basis for malignant transformation of BHK cells by chemical carcinogens. *Nature (London)*, **264**, 722
29. Ishii, Y., Elliott, J. A., Mishra, N. K. and Lieberman, M. W. (1977). Quantitative studies of transformation by chemical carcinogens and ultraviolet radiation using a subclone of BHK 21 Clone 13 Syrian hamster cells. *Cancer Res.*, **37**, 2023
30. Sugimura, T., Kawachi, T. Matsushima, T. Nagao, M., Sato, S. and Yahagi, T. (1977). A critical review of submammalian systems for mutagen detection. In: D. Scott, B. A. Bridges and G. H. Sobels (eds.). *Progress in Genetic Toxicology* pp. 126–154 Amsterdam: Elsevier Biomedical Press/North-Holland
31. Nagao, M., Yahagi, T. Honda, M. Seino, Y. Matsushima, T. and Sugimura, T. (1977). Demonstration of mutagenicity of aniline and o-toluidine by norharman. *Proc. Jpn. Acad.*, **53**, 34
32. Nagao, M., Yahagi, T., Kawachi, T. Sugimura, T. Kosuge, T. Tsuji, K., Wakabayashi, K. Mizusaki, S. and Matsumototo, T. (1977). Comutagenic action of norharman and harman. *Proc. Jpn. Acad.*, **53**, 95
33. Ashby, J., Styles, J. A., Anderson, Diana and Paton, D. (1978). Saccharin: an epigenetic carcinogen/mutagen? *Food Cosmet. Toxicol.*, **16**, 95

9

Implications of carcinogenicity
John Ashby

INTRODUCTION

The major implication of discovering a new chemical carcinogen, whether synthetic or natural, is that it may present a carcinogenic risk to exposed populations. Only in cases where a significant manufacturing or environmental exposure to that chemical exists will a possible carcinogenic hazard exist. It is therefore essential that a system of hazard assessment should be devised. The above approach assumes that chemical carcinogens are easily and clearly definable – but such, of course, is not the case. One of the major causes of confusion in this area is due to a fear felt by many that insufficient or circumstantial evidence of carcinogenicity will be used to stimulate the response usually reserved for established carcinogens. For example, few people would disagree with attempts to remove a recognizable source of potential hazard such as dimethylnitrosamine from drinking water, but many would question whether abrupt action should be taken on finding that the skin of broiled fish contains pyrolysis products mutagenic to *Salmonella typhimurium*.

The results of lifetime studies in animals are usually taken as the surest indication of carcinogenicity, but even this technique often gives inconclusive results. Quite apart from the cases where it is unclear if a genuine carcinogenic effect has been produced there are two more fundamental concerns. The first is that the degree of carcinogenicity of a chemical is often dependent upon such variables as the species, strain, age, sex, diet and route of exposure of the test animal. These uncertainties are generally accepted because it is not usually possible to predict which set of experimental conditions most closely resemble those affecting man.

The second concern is that carcinogenicity data generated for a chemical using levels of exposure far in excess of those likely to be encountered by man, and via an effective but perhaps unrepresentative route of administration, may be defining a carcinogenic potential unlikely to be realized under the actual conditions of human exposure.

Until recently the only method of recognizing a potential human carcinogen was to demonstrate a carcinogenic effect for that chemical in animals. On occasions, this approach was supplemented by structural analysis; the visual recognition of potential carcinogens by chemical structure. For example, dimethoxybenzidine(I) could be considered as a possible carcinogen simply by virtue of its structural similarity to the carcinogen benzidine(II) (see below).

IN VITRO TESTS FOR CARCINOGENICITY

The advent of short-term in vitro 'carcinogenicity' assays has presented the prospect of a short-cut to carcinogen definition, and thereby challenged the position previously held by long-term animal tests. Many in vitro carcinogenicity assays are now available, most of which are based upon either bacterial mutation or mammalian cell transformation effects, and several provide an impressive correlation between carcinogenicity and the endpoint of the assay. If these tests were completely reliable (i.e. 100% predictive of carcinogenic activity) there would be few remaining problems, but they are not. Incorrect predictions are made, both false-positive and false-negative, and although these appear to be few they cannot be neglected.

The incorrect predictions made by in vitro assays, which are often minimized by supporters and emphasized by opponents of such tests, should be approached logically. First, however, it is necessary to emphasize

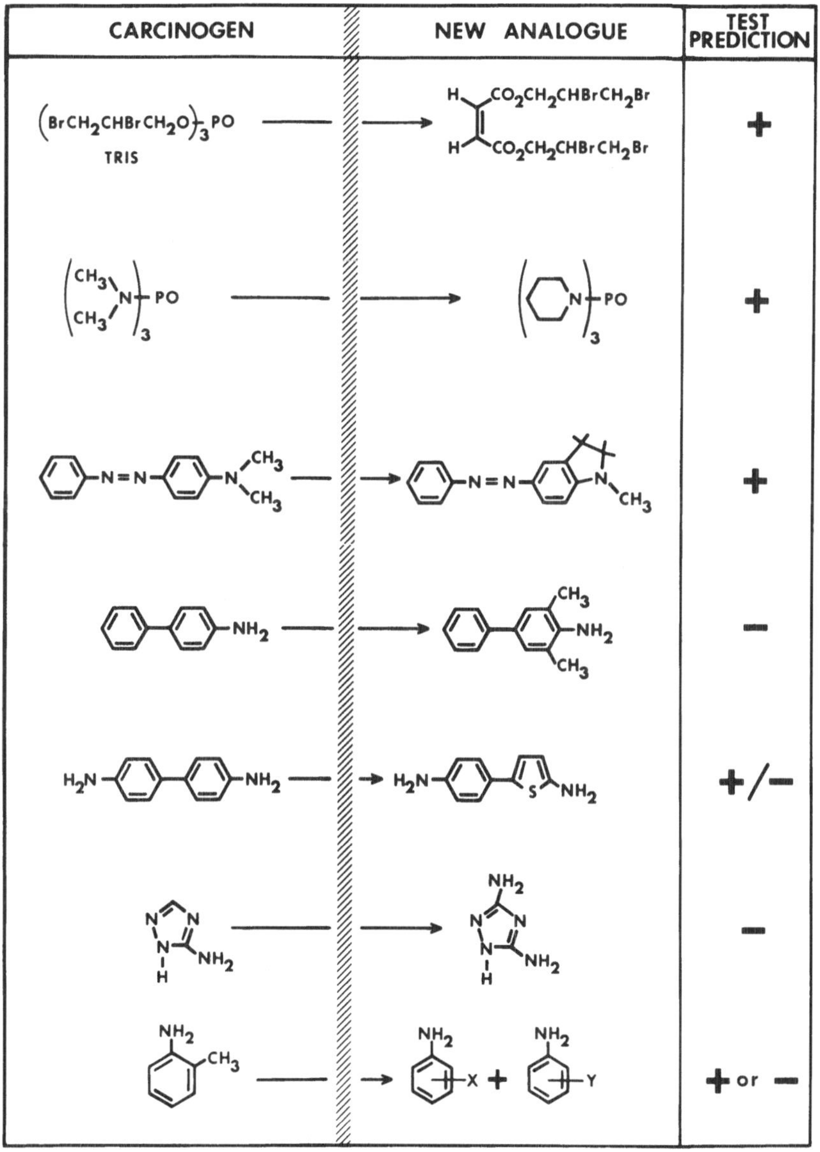

Figure 9.1 *In vitro* test predictions of possible carcinogenicity produced for the novel analogues shown on the right of the established carcinogens listed

the immense usefulness of these tests, as they undoubtedly represent a major advance in the study of potential carcinogens.

Figure 9.1 lists the type of question that these assays can answer rapidly. Compounds on the left are established carcinogens, and those on the right, compounds structurally related to them but of unknown carcinogenicity. The final column lists the predictions of activity made by *in vitro* assays, and several similar predictions have now been confirmed *in vivo*. If such predictions are assessed within the total context of biochemical, pharmacokinetic and chemical considerations, a confident assessment of the carcinogenicity of such test compounds can be made. This is indeed progress, considering that not long ago several years and large amounts of money would have had to be expended in obtaining similar answers from animal studies.

Faced with such impressive and potentially valuable assays the relevant issue is perhaps 'implications of short-term tests' rather than 'implications of carcinogenicity'. All that separates these two phrases are the 'false predictions', so a study of how and why the latter arise may be profitable.

The advantages to be gained by directly studying false predictions are several. The first is that when we know why such mistakes are made we will be in a better position to anticipate and to avoid similar mistakes in future.

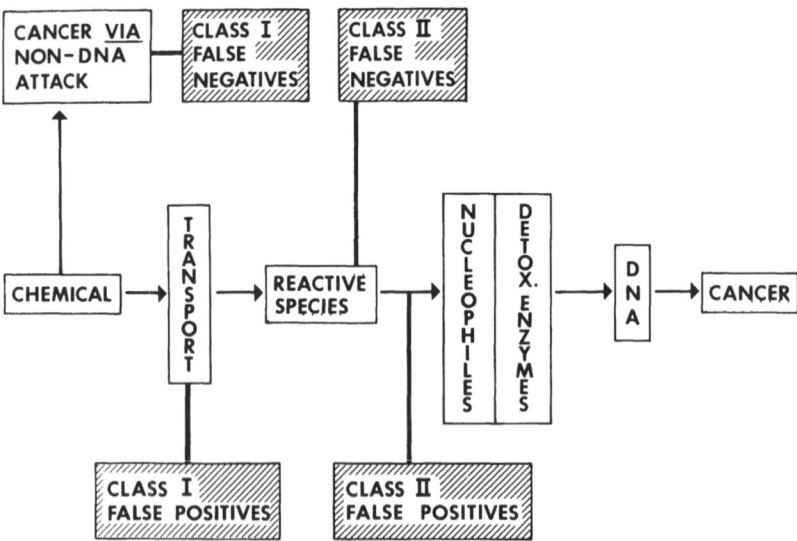

Figure 9.2   Simplified diagram of the progress of a chemical from administration *in vivo* to tumour production. The areas in which false results could arise are shown as cross-hatched boxes

Secondly, a knowledge of these mistakes will enable a clearer picture to be drawn of what validation figures of ~90% predictivity really mean. Why, for example, are these assays not 100% predictive and could they appear to be of low predictivity if different chemicals were to be studied?

Based upon theoretical, conceptual and experimental considerations, at least four types of 'false' predictions can be anticipated, the genesis of which is shown diagrammatically in Figure 9.2 and described below.

Class I false-negatives

The possibility that some carcinogens may elicit their effect *via* a non-mutagenic mechanism has been discussed for many years and has still not been finally resolved. Clearly, a carcinogen which causes cancer without

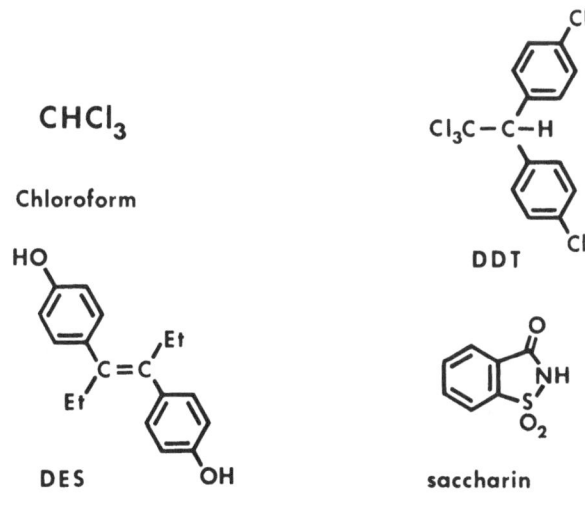

Figure 9.3 Carcinogens which may give false-negative results in *in vitro* assays due to the fact that they may produce cancer *via* a mechanism which does not require an initial chemical attack on DNA (see Figure 9.2 for key)

reacting with the DNA of cells will be negative in any assay based on DNA modification. Some possible examples of this type of compound are shown in Figure 9.3. These compounds can elicit tumours in some experimental animals under some conditions of testing, but they are negative in most of the mutation-based assays. If these compounds truly operate by an *epigenetic* mechanism no amount of technical modification of a mutation-based test will ensure their detection. Assays with some form of cellular disturbance as their endpoint, as opposed to genetic change, may be best equipped to detect such compounds.

Class II false-negatives

Most carcinogens/mutagens require to be transformed into active (electrophilic) species before they can react with DNA. In a living animal this activation is achieved at various metabolic centres, such as the liver. When a compound is tested *in vitro*, metabolic activation is simulated with a subfraction of an homogenate of rat liver, the S-9 mix.

For compounds which require several separate steps to achieve their activation it is to be expected that the S-9 mix will not always exactly recreate the enzyme activities and balances of the liver *in vivo*. For example, a key activation enzyme may be absent from the S-9 mix or particular deactivation enzymes may be over-represented. In such cases the S-9 mix may be incapable of generating the necessary dynamic balance of active species needed to inflict the required damage upon DNA; they will therefore appear to be inactive.

This type of false-negative chemical is characterized by giving an erratic or negative response *in vitro*. Such compounds can, or should be able to give a positive response *in vitro*, but such a response cannot always be reproduced under apparently identical conditions. Some examples of compounds within this category are shown in Figure 9.4. These compounds present the added problem that it would, in most cases, be possible technically to modify the test system such that they would be routinely detected as positive, but although this seems to be desirable it implies both that a standard test protocol is not practical and that the required protocol changes can be anticipated for all unknown test compounds, which is unlikely. Figure 9.5 shows results obtained in the Styles cell transformation assay for a series of derivatives of the carcinogen HMPA. Reproducibly positive or reproducibly negative results can be obtained simply by making changes to the S-9 activation system, thereby illustrating the principles discussed above. HMPA itself is usually negative in the *Salmonella* assay.

Class II False Negatives (activation).

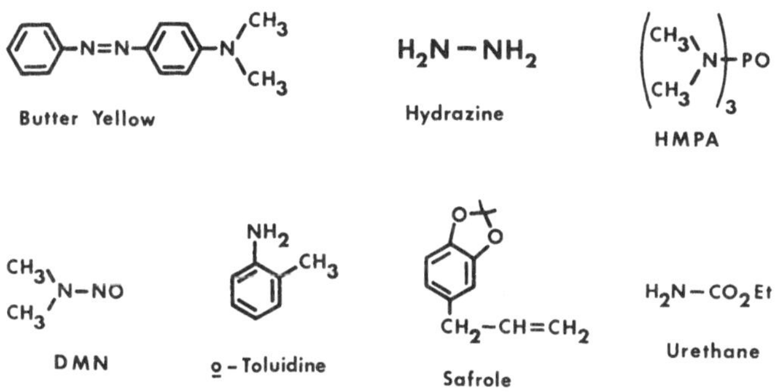
Butter Yellow
Hydrazine
HMPA
DMN
o - Toluidine
Safrole
Urethane

Figure 9.4 Carcinogens whose negative response *in vitro* is probably associated with a failure of the *in vitro* activation system (S-9 mix) to correctly simulate metabolism *in vivo*

COMPOUND / EXPERIMENT		CLASS + VE CONTROL: $[(CH_3)_2N]_3P{=}O$ (HMPA)	$[(CH_3)_2N]_3P$	$[(CH_3)_2N]_3P{=}S$	$[O(CH_2CH_2)_2N]_3P{=}S$	$[(CH_2)_5N]_3P{=}O$	$EtO{-}P(O)(N(CH_2CH_2)_2O){-}OEt$ (DEMPA)	CLASS − VE CONTROL: $[PhNH]_3P{=}O$
10 µl S−9 MIX 1:9	1	+	+	−	−	−	−	−
	2	+	+	−	−	−	−	−
50 µl S−9 MIX 1:1	3	+	+	+	+	+	+	−
	4	+	+	+	+	+	+	−

Figure 9.5 *In vitro* response obtained for a series of potential carcinogens related to the rodent carcinogen hexamethylphosphoramide (HMPA). The results demonstrate that changes to the S-9 mix (activation system) can critically affect the *in vitro* response obtained (results generated in the Styles cell transformation assay)

False-positive results

The identification of false-positive results present a greater problem than do false-negative results. This is primarily due to the absence or inadequacy of supportive long-term animal data. Nonetheless, such results are certain to exist and an attempt is made below to delineate whence they might come

Class I false-positives

The basic reason for expecting disagreements of this type is that *in vitro* tests present their DNA in a very exposed environment compared to that of the DNA of mammals. Thus, methyl orange (Figure 9.6) a fairly well-

Class I. **False Positives** (Transport)

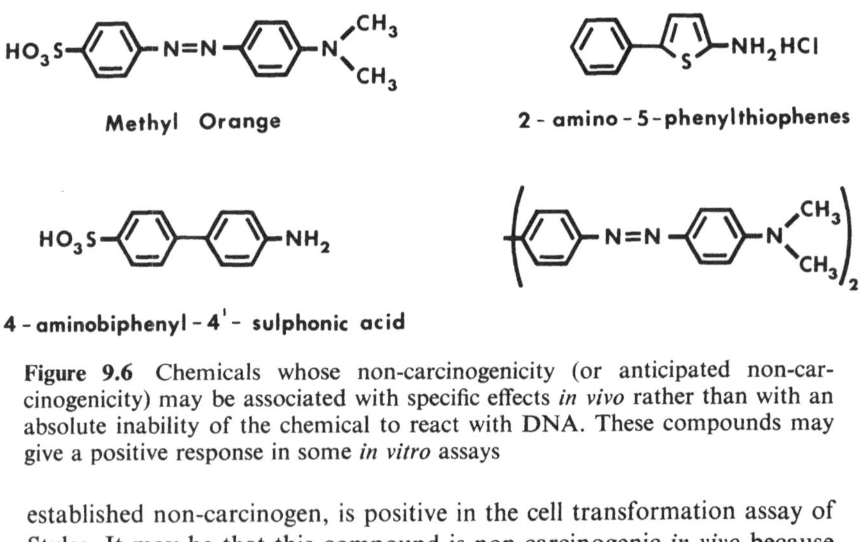

Methyl Orange

2 - amino - 5 - phenylthiophenes

4 - aminobiphenyl - 4'- sulphonic acid

Figure 9.6 Chemicals whose non-carcinogenicity (or anticipated non-carcinogenicity) may be associated with specific effects *in vivo* rather than with an absolute inability of the chemical to react with DNA. These compounds may give a positive response in some *in vitro* assays

established non-carcinogen, is positive in the cell transformation assay of Styles. It may be that this compound is non-carcinogenic *in vivo* because the polar and lipophobic sulphonic acid group imposes a distribution profile on this chemical in a living animal which prevents the potentially DNA-reactive–NMe$_2$ group from reaching and interacting chemically with DNA.

In an *in vitro* test such distribution barriers are weakened or absent, so the molecule may be forced 'unnaturally' into contact with DNA, and when this happens a positive response will be obtained. The basis of this rather diffuse class lies in the concept that 'A pulmonary carcinogen which never comes into contact with the lungs of a living animal is not a pulmonary carcinogen'. Specific animal studies will be required to estimate the importance of this group. Some other possible examples of this class of chemicals are shown in Figure 9.6.

Class II false-positives

This class arises from an extension of the above considerations, that is, that *in vitro* tests may fail to anticipate correctly the deactivation pathways acting on a reactive chemical *in vivo*. Some possible examples of chemicals within this class are shown in Figure 9.7 and the underlying principle for their giving false results is shown diagrammatically in Figure 9.8.

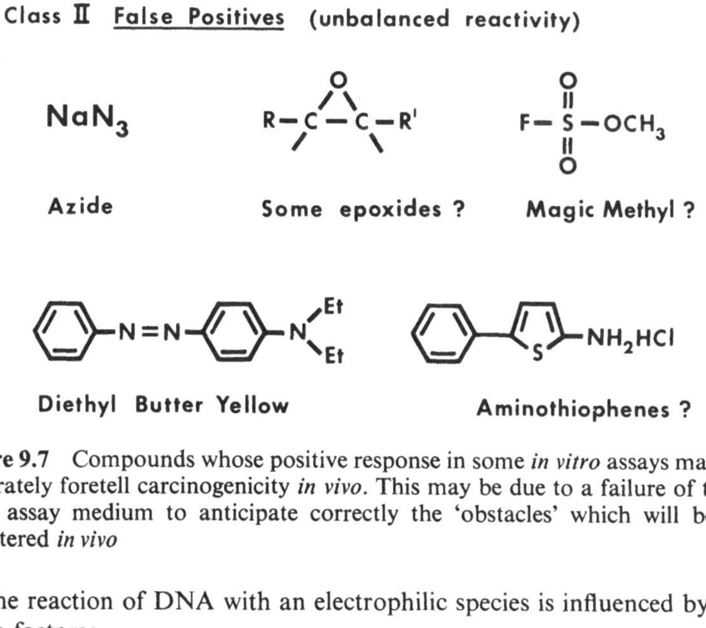

Class II False Positives (unbalanced reactivity)

NaN₃

Azide

Some epoxides ?

Magic Methyl ?

Diethyl Butter Yellow

Aminothiophenes ?

Figure 9.7   Compounds whose positive response in some *in vitro* assays may not accurately foretell carcinogenicity *in vivo*. This may be due to a failure of the *in vitro* assay medium to anticipate correctly the 'obstacles' which will be encountered *in vivo*

The reaction of DNA with an electrophilic species is influenced by two main factors:

1. The *inherent* reactivity of the chemical to DNA; this will be variable from chemical to chemical and will be dependent upon the substitution pattern and steric effects associated with each particular chemical.

2. The *attractiveness* of nuclear DNA to the reactive species as compared with competing nucleophiles (such as water, SH and NH_2 groups) and competing deactivating enzymes.

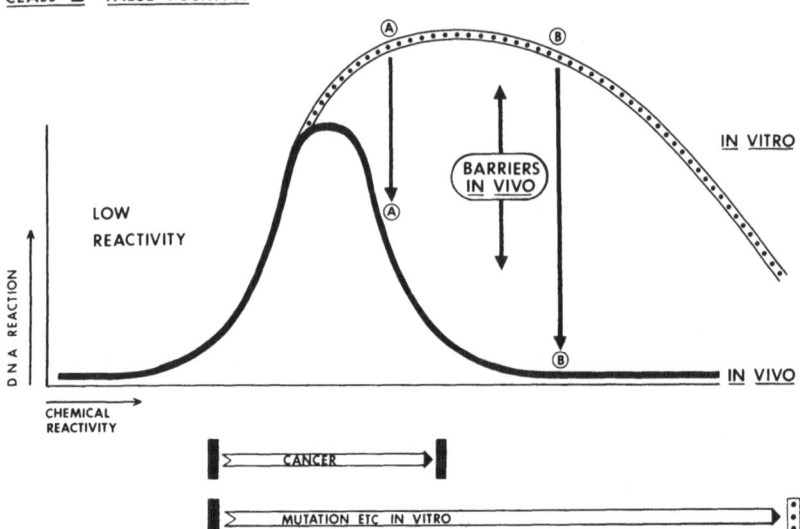

CLASS II FALSE POSITIVES

Figure 9.8   Illustration of how carcinogenicity may be related to 'optimum' chemical reactivity (electrophilicity) and how mutagenicity etc. *in vitro* may respond to a much larger range of chemical reactivity

If these two factors are related to an animal carcinogenicity study it becomes clear that within a given chemical class of potential carcinogens (such as alkylating agents) there will be a smooth transition, with changes in chemical structure, from complete inactivity to DNA, through optimum reactivity to DNA, and finally to non-reactivity to DNA. The latter stage will be reached when the chemical is *so* reactive to other nucleophiles that it cannot exist for a long enough time to complete the hazardous journey to intranuclear DNA.

This smooth transition *in vivo* is represented in Figure 9.8 by the continuous curve. The dotted extension curve represents activity *in vitro*. Faced with a diminished number of biological hurdles, activity *in vitro* may outstretch activity *in vivo*. Therefore *in vitro* tests might indicate that both compounds (A) and (B) are active, yet when the natural *in vivo* obstacles are imposed upon these activities compound (B) might dissipate its DNA reactivity, and thereby appear as non-carcinogenic, whilst the activity of compound (A) may only be attenuated, and it will therefore appear to be carcinogenic. It may be possible to add a specific nucleophile, such as piperidine, to the S-9 mix which would make a 'superactive' alkylating agent such as magic methyl (FSO_3Me, suggested to be point (B) in Figure 9.8) appear as negative *in vitro* whilst leaving as positive a carcinogenic alkylating agent of medium activity such as dimethyl sulphate [$(CH_3O)_2SO_2$] (suggested to be point (A) in Figure 9.8). In this way conditions *in vitro* could be regulated to those occurring *in vivo* by means of titrating the S-9 mix to a given 'piperidine figure'. This class of result is epitomized by the concept that 'An expert pearl-fisher who cannot swim underwater is no pearl-fisher at all'. It was recently observed that the addition of cysteine to the medium of the Ames assay can profoundly reduce the mutagenic potency of some mutagens, and this is clearly related to the above considerations.

What do predictivity figures of 90% really mean?

The real and hypothetical considerations outlined above indicate that the predictivity figure associated with an *in vitro* assay will be dependent upon the type of chemical chosen for the test. If long-term animal testing facilities are used only to confirm the predictions made by *in vitro* assays for chemicals such as dimethylsulphate and sugar then these assays will appear to be highly predictive of carcinogenicity. This is because the activity of such compounds could have been correctly anticipated via chemical and biochemical considerations.

At the other extreme, if 'problem' compounds and their structural analogues such as those discussed above are pursued, these tests may well appear to be completely non-predictive of carcinogenicity (see Table 9.1). Alternatively, the study of such compounds might confirm the suggestion

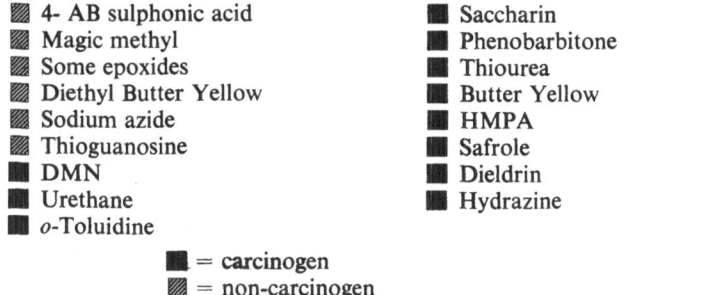

Table 9.1   Validation to show *in vitro* tests ~ 0 % predictive*

Methyl orange	Chloroform
Aminothiophenes	DDT
Bis-Butter Yellow	DES
4- AB sulphonic acid	Saccharin
Magic methyl	Phenobarbitone
Some epoxides	Thiourea
Diethyl Butter Yellow	Butter Yellow
Sodium azide	HMPA
Thioguanosine	Safrole
DMN	Dieldrin
Urethane	Hydrazine
o-Toluidine	

= carcinogen
= non-carcinogen

* A ~ 100% predictive study would be even easier to design

that the present 'false' predictions of *in vitro* assays would disappear if these compounds were to be adequately tested *in vivo*. Should this prove true these assays would then be established as capable of replacing animal studies. Either way, such studies would be worth while.

CARCINOGENIC INHIBITION AND POTENTIATION

The problems which already have been or predictably could be encountered with *in vitro* assays are already well established in the field of animal carcinogenicity. For example, it is well known that the co-administration of certain chemicals (usually competing nucleophiles, specific enzyme poisons or free-radical scavengers) with a carcinogen can reduce or abolish the carcinogenicity of the latter. A specific example is afforded by the carcinogenicity of 2-acetylaminofluorene (2-AAF)(III) which is dramatically reduced if acetanilide(IV), a non-carcinogen, is administered with it (see below). This effect has been associated with the ability of acetanilide to poison the N→O transacetylase enzyme system critical to the metabolic activation of 2AAF as a carcinogen.

(III)   (IV)

The related topic of carcinogenic potentiation, or synergism, will probably be governed by similar laws, although this subject has not yet been studied in detail. An indication that carcinogenic synergism *may* be an important consideration when assessing the hazard from human exposure to chemicals is afforded by the following *in vivo/in vitro* observations.

The carcinogenic potency of the rat-liver carcinogen Butter Yellow(V) is heavily dependent upon the levels of the deactivating azoreductase enzymes present in the liver of the test animal. These in turn are dependent on the riboflavin content of the diet of the test animal. Thus, when these levels are low, Butter Yellow appears to be a moderately potent carcinogen, but when they are high it appears to be almost non-carcinogenic. The metabolic interconversions observed for this chemical (see Figure 9.9)

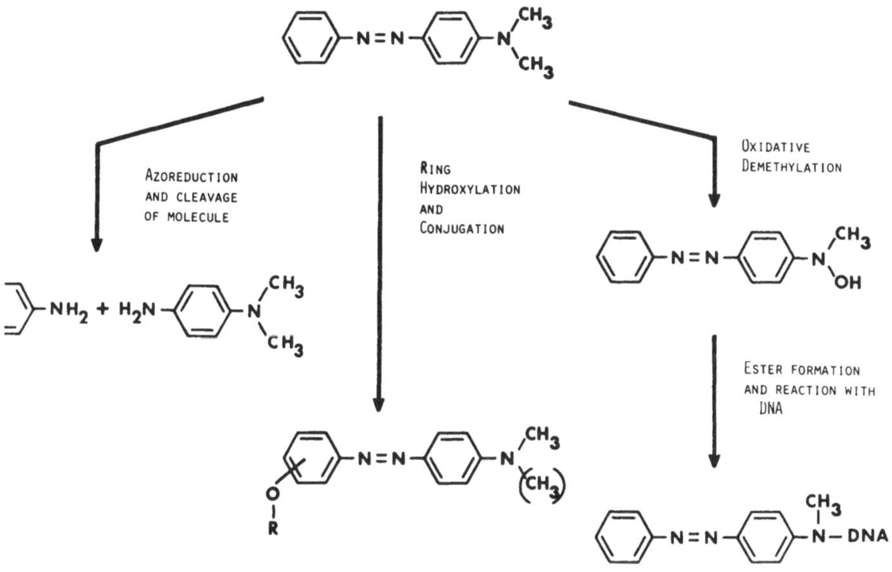

Figure 9.9 Metabolism (based on both *in vivo* and *in vitro* studies) of 4-dimethylaminoazobenzene (Butter Yellow)

enable the above variations to be explained. In order for Butter Yellow to react with DNA, the $-NMe_2$ group must be enzymically transformed whilst the remainder of the molecule remains intact. Acting against this activation pathway are two deactivating pathways namely splitting of the

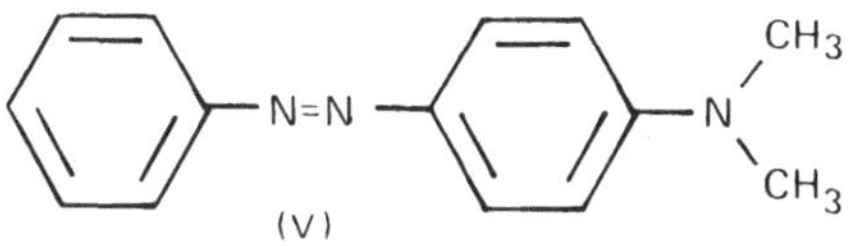

(V)

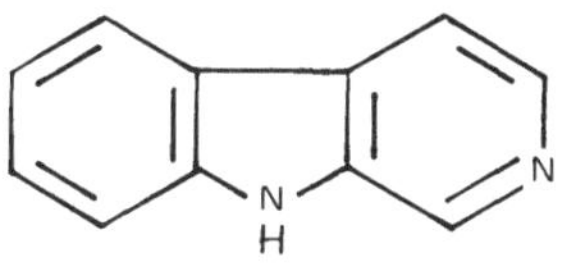

(VI)

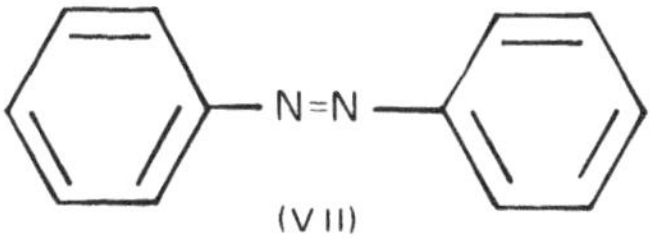

(VII)

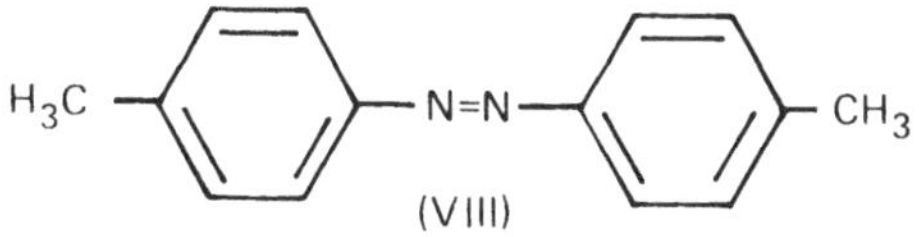

(VIII)

molecule via azoreductase enzymes, and ring-hydroxylation and con-
jugation of the intact molecule. The net activation of DAB obtained (and
thereby the net carcinogenicity observed?) will depend upon the balance of
activation and deactivation, a balance which in this case is dependent
upon the riboflavin content of the diet of the test animal. It has been
observed that the *in vitro* response given by this chemical can be increased
by the addition of the non-mutagen norharman(VI) to the assay medium.
It is therefore possible that the latter is inhibiting, either competitively or
non-competitively, the ring-hydroxylation enzyme system which de-
activates Butter Yellow, thereby increasing its apparent potency *in vitro*
(Figure 9.10). It could equally be anticipated that 'diversion' of the

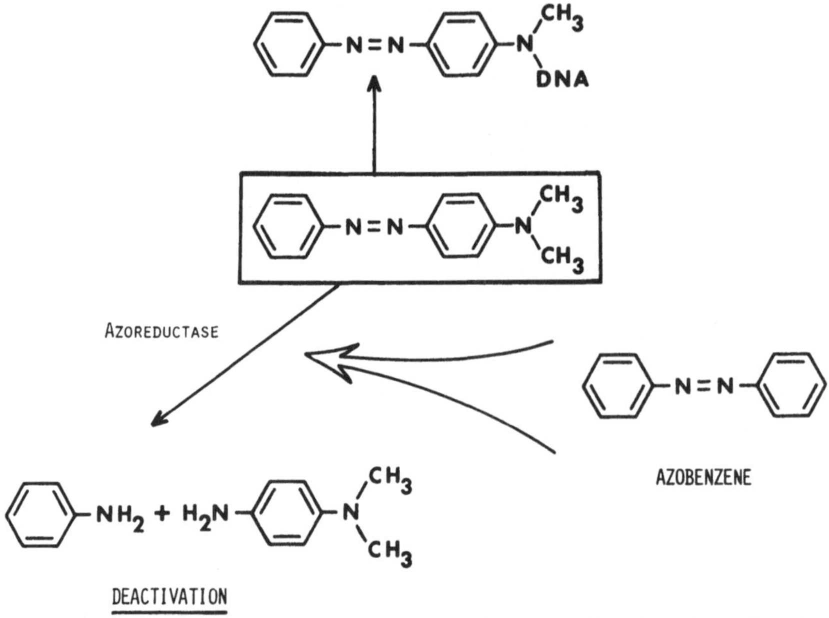

Figure 9.10 Illustration of how norharman is suggested to interfere with the
detoxification of Butter Yellow via competitive interaction with the ring-hydroxylation detoxification enzyme system of the S-9 mix (from Nagao *et al.* (1977)

azoreductase enzyme system with a suitable competitive substrate, such as
the non-carcinogen azobenzene(VII), would also increase the net activation of Butter Yellow (Figure 9.11).

Such an effect has been demonstrated *in vitro* using the Styles cell
transformation assay. Figure 9.12 shows the negative response given by
azobenzene (AB), and the positive response given by Butter Yellow (BY)
when tested alone. The third response is that given by a 1:1 mixture of

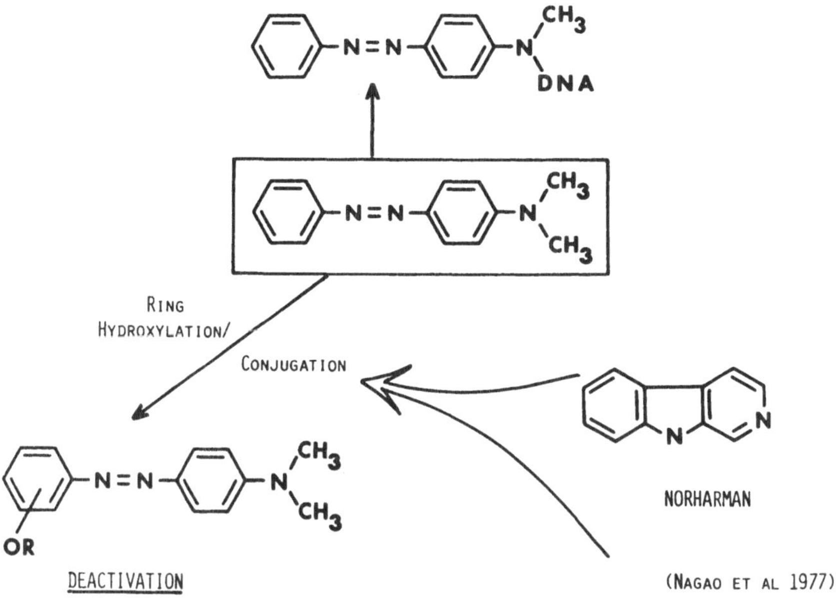

Figure 9.11   Illustration of how azobenzene is suggested to interfere with the detoxification of Butter Yellow via competitive interaction with the azoreductase detoxification enzyme system of the S-9 mix

azobenzene and Butter Yellow (AB + BY) and it shows a 25-fold increase in the potency of Butter Yellow as a cell-transforming agent *in vitro*. This apparent demonstration of synergism *in vitro* should not be translated into synergism *in vivo* too readily. For example, the only relevant experiment conducted *in vivo* concerns the co-administration of Butter Yellow(V) and 4,4-dimethylazobenzene(VIII). In this case, which may have been expected to follow the *in vitro* azobenzene experiment referred to above, a marked protective affect was observed, tumour appearance being delayed as compared to Butter Yellow. Nonetheless, carcinogenic potentiation or synergism experiments conducted *in vivo* are bound to be realized in some cases.

The considerations developed throughout this article have been summarized in Figure 9.13. This figure enables the phrase *potential carcinogen* to be accurately defined and suggests that there may be two classes of non-carcinogens recorded in the literature: the first, a group of *absolute* non-carcinogens, and the second, compounds which are potential carcinogens but which have so far *failed* to produce a carcinogenic effect *in vivo*. Chemicals within the latter group could possibly be induced to produce

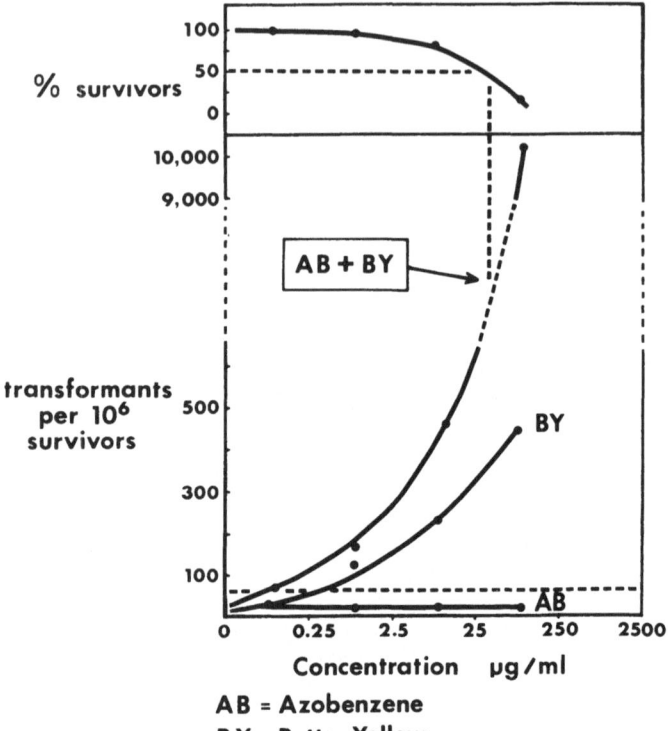

Figure 9.12 Response given by the non-carcinogen azobenzene (AB), the carcinogen Butter Yellow (BY) and a 1:1 mixture of azobenzene + Butter Yellow (AB+BY) in the Styles cell transformation assay

tumours by the appropriate choice of animal species and strain, or diet, etc. These arguments cast some doubt on the historical concept of *absolute* carcinogens and non-carcinogens but this should not be abandoned too readily, at least not until an alternative basis can be found upon which to form decisions concerning the potential human hazard presented by exposure to a given chemical.

The above reasoning also leads to the hypothesis that many compounds may be chemically equipped and theoretically able to cause cancer under individually optimized metabolic circumstances, but only a proportion of these may be capable of inducing tumours under the metabolic conditions of an *in vivo* study. If this is the case, a dilemma is posed by the fact that *in vitro* carcinogenicity assays detect the *potential* rather than the *ability* of a chemical to cause cancer *in vivo*. As the number of compounds in the former category may be significantly larger than those in the latter, some

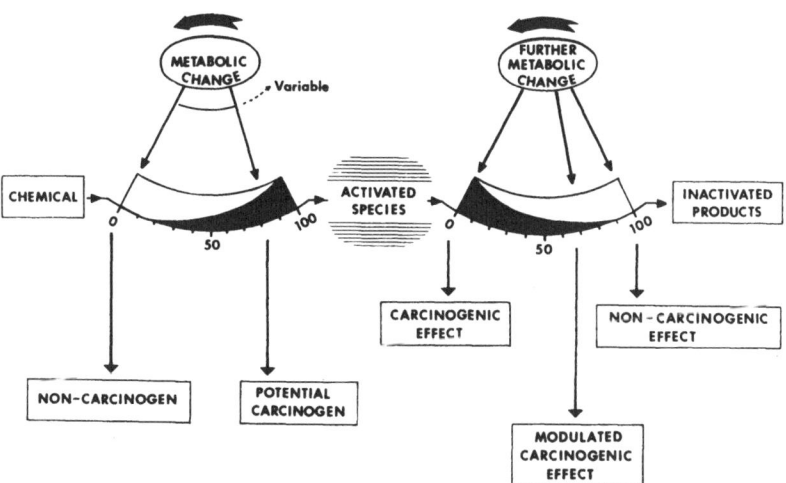

Figure 9.13 Diagrammatic representation of the moderating effects produced by competitive metabolic pathways on the carcinogenicity of a compound. The starting compound is assumed not to be a direct-acting carcinogen. In such cases the compound would be placed directly in the central box. The position of the indicator in each dial could affect the *in vitro* response given by a compound. The exact indicator positions will be influenced by firstly, the diet, sex, age, species and strain of the test animal, and dose-levels employed in an *in vivo* study, and secondly, the method of induction, preparation and storage of the liver S-9 mix used in an *in vitro* assay and the presence of competitive enzyme substrates, both *in vivo* and *in vitro*

attention should be given to what is inferred from the results of such *in vitro* assays. In particular, the following question should be answered: are carcinogen-screening programmes designed to protect the majority of a population from exposure to easily demonstrable animal carcinogens, or are they also to be used to protect all metabolically idiosyncratic minorities of a population from each and every possible carcinogen? (The metabolic differences of these subgroups may be environmentally or genetically determined.) The existence of such sub-groups is probably evidenced by the non-uniform incidence of tumours generally observed when either animals or humans are exposed to chemical carcinogens. The answer to the above question will determine whether the enzyme profile of the S-9 liver fraction used in *in vitro* assays should be regulated, as far as is possible, to that encountered by a chemical in the liver of an average man, or if it is to be individually optimized, perhaps as a 'cocktail' of individually purified enzymes, to give the maximum chance of obtaining a positive response for each compound.

In summary, carcinogenic and mutagenic effects are complex phenomena. This complexity will of necessity be increased by the need to study such effects in lower organisms and then extrapolate such results to man. We will never be able to protect *everybody* from every possible hazard, so a compromise must be reached. This compromise can only be arrived at after a balanced consideration of the following factors.

1. Likely human exposure to the chemical.
2. The predictions of *in vitro* carcinogenicity tests.
3. Chemical, biochemical and pharmacokinetic considerations which will help to estimate the *likelihood* of expression in man of effects observed *in vitro*.

4. The protective defences (non-critical nucleophiles, detoxification enzymes, immunosurveillance mechanisms, etc.) of animals and man. To swamp these defences in an animal carcinogenicity or mutagenicity study, by using very high exposure levels, may be to generate data which will be of little or no value for extrapolating to an average man, with intact defences, at low levels of exposure.

To realize the above objectives, specific carcinogenicity studies will be needed to evaluate the nature and likely frequency of false predictions made by *in vitro* tests. Further, in order that general credibility in short-term tests should be retained, a *justification* for any new test, and perhaps some of the recently announced ones, should be clearly given. It is perhaps no longer justifiable to develop a new assay (for example a new strain of *E. coli* or of *S. typhimurium*, etc.) and *then* decide if it *could* be useful. Rather, new tests should be sought which fill a gap left by the available tests. A short-term test which *clearly* and *reliably* detects saccharin or DDT as positive may be of more immediate value than yet another test which detects, in common with most other tests, benzo(a)pyrene and Aflatoxin B_1 as positive. For example, specific enzyme changes have recently been associated with exposure of animals to both saccharin and dieldrin. If pursued, these may form the basis of a test for the carcinogenicity of such agents.

Acknowledgement

The biological data shown in Figures 9.5 and 9.12 were generated by Dr J. A. Styles using his own cell transformation assay. I also wish to thank the *British Journal of Cancer* for granting permission to reproduce Figures 9.5, 9.9, 9.12 and 9.15, for all of which they hold the copyright.

References

To ease the flow of this article it has not been specifically referenced. However, all of the work discussed, both from our laboratory and from those of others, has been described and referenced in detail in the following publications:

1. Ashby, J., Styles, J. A. and Paton, D. (1978). *In vitro* evaluation of some derivatives of the carcinogen butter yellow: implications for environmental screening. *Bri. J. Cancer*, **38**, 34
2. Ashby, J. and Styles, J. A. (1978). Comutagenicity, competitive enzyme substrates, and *in vitro* carcinogenicity assays. *Mutat. Res.*, **54**, 105
3. Ashby, J., Styles, J. A., Anderson, D. and Paton, D. (1978). Saccharin: An epigenetic carcinogen/mutagen? *Food and Cosmet. Toxicol.*, **16**, 95
4. Ashby, J. Styles, J. A. and Paton, D. (1978). Potentially carcinogenic analogues of the carcinogen hexamethylphosphoramide (HMPA). *Br. J. Cancer*, **38**, 34
5. Ashby, J., Anderson, D. and Styles, J. A. (1978). The potential carcinogenicity of methyl fluorosulphonate (CH_3OSO_2F; magic methyl). *Mutat. Res.*, **51**, 285
6. Ashby, J. and Purchase, I. F. H. (1977). The selection of appropriate chemical class controls for use with short-term tests for potential carcinogenicity. *Ann. Occup. Hygiene*, **20**, 297
7. Ashby, J., Styles, J. A. and Anderson, D. (1977). Selection of an *in vitro* carcinogenicity test for derivatives of the carcinogen hexamethylphosphoramide. *Br. J. Cancer*, **36**, 564
8. Ashby, J. and Styles, J. A., (1978). Does carcinogenic potency correlate with mutagenic potency in the Ames assay? *Nature (London)*, **271**, 452, and subsequent correspondence *Nature (London)*, **274**, 19
9. Ashby, J., Anderson, D. Styles, J. A. and Paton, D. (1978). Thiophene analogues of the carcinogens benzidine and 4-aminobiphenyl: evaluation *in vitro*, *Br. J. Cancer*, **38**, 521
10. Purchase, I. F. H., Longstaff, E., Ashby, J., Styles, J. A., Anderson, D. Lefevre, P. A., and Westwood, F. R. (1978). *Br. J. Cancer*, 873 (Appendix I), 904
11. Crabtree, H. G. (1955). Retardation of azo-carcinogenesis by non-carcinogenic azo-compounds. *Br. J. Cancer*, **9**, 310
12. Wattenberg, L. W. (1978). Inhibitors of chemical carcinogenesis. *Adv. Cancer Res.*, **26**, 197
13. Moriya, M., Kato, K. and Shirasu, Y. (1978). Effects of cysteine and a liver metabolic activation system on the activities of mutagenic pesticides. *Mutat. Res.*, **57**, 259
14. Rosin, M. P. and Stich, H. F. (1978). The inhibitory effect of cysteine on the mutagenic activities of several carcinogens. *Mutat. Res.*, **54**, 73
15. Yamato, R. S., Williams, G. M., Richardson, H. L., Weisburger, E. K. and Weisburger, J. H. (1973). Effects of *p*-hydroxyacetanilide on liver cancer induction by *N*-hydroxy-*N*-2-fluorenylacetamide. *Cancer Res.*, **33**, 154

184   MUTAGENESIS IN SUB-MAMMALIAN SYSTEMS

16. Vesely, D. L. and Levy, G. S. (1978). Saccharin inhibits guanylate cyclase activity – possible relationship to carcinogenesis. *Biochem. Biophys. Res. Commun.*, **81,** 1384
17. Kohli, K. K. and Venkitasubramanian, T. A. (1978). Effect of dieldrin toxicity on pyridine nucleotides and activities of NADH and NADPH oxidase in rat liver. *Chem. Biol. Interact.*, **21,** 337

Discussion

Chairman: Professor D. Parke

Professor L. EHRENBERG (Stockholm): Dr Dean raises an important point. There are situations of accidental exposure – for example in industry – to a chemical where other factors could be used to calculate the dose that had been received, and where some kind of standard could be evolved and through it what was found in the outer environment could later be related. The real problem has turned out to be the industry's unwillingness to provide access to the records dealing with the exposure. I know from my own experience of one case in the US in 1974, and one case in Great Britain in 1975, of heavy exposure to a chemical where such a situation could have arisen – in both cases around 30 workers were involved, and there was no possibility of access to the workers for that kind of study. This is the kind of problem that has to be solved on some level.

Dr B. J. DEAN (Sittingbourne): I fully agree. We did a very large survey of a population of about two or three hundred mothers and their children some 10 years ago – mothers who had previously taken oral contraceptives and then come off them to get pregnant. Looking at it later, it was significant how predictive it had been of the oestrogens and the progestogens which had been indicted by subsequent studies in dogs and primates. There were two cases – two babies that had chromosomal abnormalities, and when we looked into the family history we found that both the fathers were chemical workers. That bears out both the Professor's points.

Mr N. J. Van ABBE (Leatherhead): Perhaps it is worth going back to an incident which I would call the aerosol adhesives fiasco, whereby some apparently false judgment on chromosome damage, and inadequate or incorrect selection of controls, has virtually completely destroyed an industry. An interesting point about that is that the fiasco emanated from the judgment of one cytogeneticist, and when the slides were re-examined by four or five others, different conclusions were reached.

How reproducible are judgments on chromosome damage?

Dr B. J. DEAN: Mr van Abbe must realize how difficult that question is to answer.

There have been surveys, obviously, where slides have been distributed to various laboratories throughout Europe, and there have been differences in interpretation. I must admit that. But from my personal experience in my own laboratory where I have four or five people who are skilled analysts – chromosome analysts – we now have a great deal of agreement. If one individual analyses a slide and finds a given percentage of aberrations, I am quite confident that I can give this same slide to another individual in the same laboratory and get virtually the same result. But there is no doubt that there is inter-laboratory variation. I am quite sure of that. These are differences in the interpretation of specific aberrations, but also differences in technique, in preparation and culture technique, and it is very difficult to know how to get over this problem. Certainly within a laboratory there should be good agreement, but between laboratories there are certainly differences.

SECTION FOUR

General Implications of Mutagenesis

10

Extrapolation of mutagenic test results to man
P. Oftedal

I am primarily concerned with a specific mutagen – radiation. However, chemical mutagen exposure can be related to radiation exposure, *radiation norms*, and direct comparisons have been made between chemicals and radiation on the basis of equivalent effects. The 'Roentgen equivalent chemical' (rec) was proposed some years ago by B. A. Bridges. Radiation exposure norms are well established and are generally accepted, and may thus be very useful in comparative situations. On the other hand, it should be realized (a) that radiation norms are in themselves frail structures and can be criticized on many points, and (b) the complexity of the chemical mutagen/carcinogen biological interaction is so great that simple and uniform solutions to the problem of standard setting are not possible as yet.

I think it is useful here to look at a simple diagram (p. 194) showing some of the elements which enter into the standard-setting procedure. This is primarily applied to radiation, but would perhaps be relevant for chemicals as well. This is the transition from scientific observation, analysis, and generalization, to the application of specific local or national standards for exposure to mutagenic/carcinogenic agents. The path runs from the base level of the scientific data, through a more-or-less detailed stepwise development to risk analysis (which is still fairly scientific in nature), to recommendations on general principles (often made by international bodies and, except for dramatic episodes, removed from detailed analysis and specific effects).

The recommendations must be translated into a set of legal rules, and now we are definitely on the national (or grouped national) level. Laws form the basis of regulations. The final step is the enforcement of the legal rules.

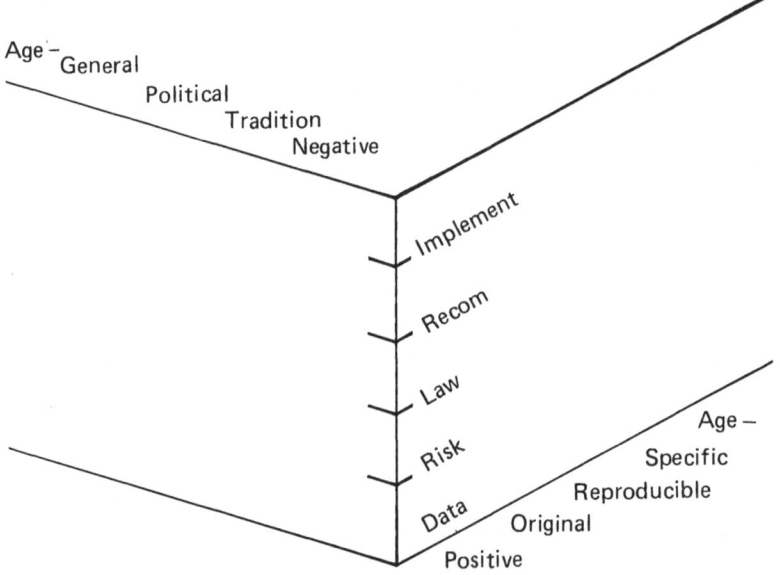

Figure 10.1   Exposure to radiation; standard setting procedure

At the levels going from the data to the regulations, we have concurrently changed our orientation from the criteria on which scientific activity is based and results judged, to a set of criteria valid for activities in society, and there are great differences. One set of criteria is as good as the other, and they are not completely without interrelationship, but they are very different.

Scientific data are judged by their merits in terms of originality, reproducibility, and specificity. They are always positive as negative findings are usually not published. This is in contrast to the social criteria applicable to the legal rules. They are based on established facts – which means they are not original. They are negative in the sense that they aim at prevention. They are tempered by a complex network of tradition and various politico-economic considerations.

Now, how can a set of standards for chemicals compare with those pertaining to radiation? Radiation exposure is governed by dose limits which are set so low that no acute effects are ever seen. From these dose limits are derived concentration and intake limits of various types. But, in addition to this, the recommendations of the International Commission on Radiological Protection (ICRP) have the important provisos that exposures should be held as low as reasonably possible, taking into consideration social and economic conditions. The exposure should furthermore be justified by the benefits of the activity. And, in addition, and again as an overriding consideration, the procedure involving exposure should be optimized. In other words, the risk from radiation should not be reduced to an absurd extent, if this leads to other risks which may be greater.

At this level – maybe 10–1000-fold below the dose limits – the radiation protection philosophy becomes as subtle and pragmatic as does the acceptable daily intakes (ADI) of chemicals, or the threshold limiting values (TLV), or maximum allowable concentrations (MAC). The ADIs are set by the Codex Alimentarius, and are formulated in a complex series of cycles spiralling between scientific working groups, central secretarial administrative treatments and political bodies, at nine different levels. A particular value becomes a rule when a certain number of governments have accepted it, so the path from the scientific to the political is obvious. The economic element enters clearly by way of the use of phrases like 'good agricultural practice', which will differ between countries and regions and which give a clear indication of the pragmatic nature of the agreement. The same applies to the TLVs, which stem largely from the United States, and which are applicable in other countries according to local needs and considerations.

As consciousness of more subtle undesirable effects of chemicals has developed, and as new chemicals have come to be used for specific biological purposes, attention has begun to be focused beyond the acute effects, and late effects have now to be considered.

With regard to radiation, the perspective of cancer on the one hand and genetic effects on the other define dangers of different types, and for which different measures are taken. For those exposed because of their occupation, the individual risk must be kept so low as to be acceptable. The risk is primarily a cancer threat, involving the individual, partly because the main part of his, or her, occupational life comes after the reproductive age, and partly because the numerical relationships are such that the individual background risk for genetic damage is not very small, while the increment over a base level is.

The other category of exposure is the population exposure, where small

individual doses still may lead to large collective doses – over great populations and long periods – and therefore to large numbers of cases of
genetic damage, though still small in relation to the natural incidence.
The *individual* cancer risk becomes very small.

With regard to the chemicals and the sub-mammalian test systems, I am
not going to make any quantitative estimates, or present any conversion
factors or acceptable limits. To my mind the time is not ready for this yet,
and may never be so. But this does not really detract from the usefulness
of these test systems. They have often been characterized as warning flags,
and this is what they are and how they should be used. In addition, they
are powerful tools for the investigation of the mechanisms involved in a
chemical's reaction with the genetic material. They are warning flags, and
should be heeded as such. But the weight of their evidence will score
differently in different situations, and this comes under the same categories
as for radiation exposure: occupational, and population exposure.

A positive test result in sub-mammalian systems for a substance predominantly used within an industry will mean mainly occupational exposure and therefore a carcinogenic risk. In that case, further tests in mammalian systems – mainly for cancer – will weigh heavily. If no confirmation
in terms of cancer induction is forthcoming, and if plausible explanations
for lack of effect can be presented, I suspect the positive test data from
sub-mammalian systems will not carry strong weight.

Captan may be a case in point, with clear mutagenic potential for occupational exposure in the agricultural professions, but with no cancer induction in test animals or epidemiological evidence from industry. The
latter is definitely not proof of non-activity, since the resolving power of
such data are very limited, but they may indicate an upper limit of uncertainty.

As a contrasting case the herbicide Amitrole may be mentioned. From
Sweden some years ago, semi-convincing epidemiological evidence from
railroad spraying teams in the 1950s related this substance to an increase
in the incidence of cancer. Subsequent tests in Finland, using a number of
sub-mammalian and chromosomal systems, have uncovered no evidence
for mutagenicity. In Norway, however, there has yet been no revoking of
the ban introduced in 1974, in spite of strong pressure from farmers who
need this agent for weed control in oats. Even the suspicion of a carcinogenic effect is sufficient to balance a whole set of negative data.

These are then occupational exposures. Positive sub-mammalian test
data would seem to be regarded as warnings, but would call for supporting
evidence from mammalian cancer tests, or from epidemiology. Changes in
working regimes and procedures would seem in order, but should only be

mildly restrictive and depend on costs. Cancer in the exposed person remains as the important endpoint.

In general exposure of the public, the situation is different in two major aspects. Firstly, much larger, more variable and more sensitive populations may be exposed. This means that any quantitative estimates developed for the occupationally exposed must be modified to accommodate an increased sensitivity. Secondly, and most important, is the change in endpoint, which must now also include genetic effects. This introduces an additional parameter of considerable biological, emotional and ethical weight.

The genetic effects in man will in all probability be of a kind for which an experimental study will never give a satisfactory negative answer at the relevant dose level. No matter how non-positive mammalian genetic experiments – dominant lethals or specific locus – may be, the doses necessary in experiments will never give relevant information regarding the effects at the exposure levels involved in planned exposures of human populations. This will be obvious if radiation is considered as an example. The doubling dose for most genetic effects in mammals appears to be about 100 rem for chronic exposures. Lifetime genetically significant doses for occupational exposure may possibly reach this order of magnitude, but the number of persons involved will be very small, and the demonstration of a statistically secure genetic effect impossible. Populations in general may receive 10–20 m rem per year, or maximally 0.5 rem per generation, which might be taken to lead, after some generations, to a 0.5% increase in some categories of genetic disease. Obviously, no epidemiology is ever going to be able to demonstrate any effects of this magnitude.

So, for genetic effects, a warning flag in the form of positive test data carry much more weight than for somatic effects, because this warning flag is probably the only signal we may get. If we return to captan for a moment, we find positive test data, and there is also a fair amount of residue in fruit. There is thus a population exposure, but the systemic fungicides are still in extensive use, mainly because of their great benefits.

The quantification of test data carries two different connotations which should be kept clearly apart. Quantification within a test system is necessary:

1) in order to establish dose-effect relationship on which interpretation of the mechanisms of mutagenesis may be based;

2) in order to compare different mutagens in one and the same test system, say, for efficiency;

3) in order to compare different test systems with the same mutagens to compare sensitivities, mechanisms, etc.

On the other hand, quantification with the aim of forming a proper risk estimate, or cost–benefit analysis, oriented towards the human situation is a different matter altogether.

A case may be made for a simple calculation to indicate a major threat to man's health or to a biological system. But the uncertainties are so many and complex that no simple answer should appear with a claim to more than a token weight. I want to mention a few of the factors which make it necessary to act *ad hoc* and specifically, rather than in general terms. Even after mechanisms are known, exposures are measured, and possible effects have been identified, standard setting of the same generality as for radiation is precluded because of the following two factors.

1. Individual variation in sensitivity. This is not the gross repair capacity differences of the XP type and the like, but difference in metabolism, in detoxification capacity, induced or obligatory, leading to synergisms at various levels. This precludes the simple addition of various loads.

2. Germ cell stage sensitivity variation, which for radiation may be of the order of 10-fold or so, but for chemicals a couple of orders or magnitude higher. With temporal differences so great, it becomes impossible to generalize over time, and any exposure has to be evaluated in the light of what has gone before, and what may come after.

The solution can be found only by a generally restrictive policy, and a careful *ad hoc* evaluation of each substance. This evaluation will be heavily weighted towards the need for demonstrating the benefits, since the costs are bound to remain unknown. And when acting on the basis of ignorance, much wider margins of safety must be carried than when acting on a basis of uncertainty.

The wide range of possible patterns of reaction puts an added responsibility on the shoulders of the researcher. It may be easy to get positive test data under a given set of conditions, but very difficult to say to what appropriate action they should lead.

11

Tests for mutagenesis from a regulatory point of view
M. H. Draper

The rapid emergence of chemical mutagenesis as a potential hazard to future generations has presented Government and other bodies with an unprecedented issue. Many Governments now accept the necessity to identify and limit the spread of chemicals with possible mutagenic properties into the human environment. It is necessary to emphasize that mutagenesis is a potential hazard in its own right because to some extent the implications of this possibility have been overshadowed by the belief that most forms of malignancy may result from somatic cell mutations; hence if a chemical is mutagenic in a test system it might also be a carcinogen.

Recent history has demonstrated that human health can be seriously affected in totally unexpected ways. The lessons learnt from these misfortunes have brought about a complete change in toxicological thinking. The fact that rubella infection can produce congenital defects reported in 1941 by Gregg[1], was the first dramatic demonstration of this. Then the thalidomide disaster occurred in the late fifties[2]. The implications of this were so unexpected and serious that the episode can be regarded as a watershed in modern toxicology. Another event of consequence was the so called Turkey X disease that resulted in the deaths of more than a hundred thousand turkeys in 1969 and which in due course drew attention to new varieties of dangerous mycotoxins (the aflatoxins among others[3]).

195

In the meantime from the early sixties onwards there was a growing awareness among biological scientists that many of the huge number of new synthetic compounds being introduced into the human environment as industrial chemicals, drugs, food additives, cosmetics or domestic aids were capable of producing mutations in simple organisms such as bacteria or the fruit fly, *Drosophila melanogaster*. Two events probably played a considerable role in persuading Government advisers that mutagenesis was yet another unsuspected toxicological hazard to the future welfare of mankind, and that steps should be taken to understand and contain it. The implications of this are that industry will be required to undertake a number of new test procedures involving radically different testing technologies. In turn the fresh insights that are arising from the fundamental nature of the mechanisms involved in genetic toxicology call for a review of toxicological testing procedures as a whole.

The first event was the discovery in 1972 that the supposedly safe food preservative AF2 (2-(2-furyl)-3-(5-nitro-2-furyl)acrylamide) which was added to a wide variety of food in Japan in 1965 was a potential mutagen. This led to a retesting for carcinogenesis and in due course malignant tumours were produced in rats and mice and hamsters. AF2 was withdrawn completely by 1974[4]. Thus it is now apparent that the Japanese nation was unwittingly exposed to what might well prove to be a potent mutagen and carcinogen in humans. The next five to ten years will confirm the reality or otherwise of the hazard to health of AF2. The second development was the enormous advance made when it was realized that the metabolic conversion of a chemical to its ultimate carcinogenic (or mutagenic) state could be brought about in a large number of chemicals by an extract of liver homogenate, the 'S9 fraction'. This contains, among other enzyme systems, the mixed function oxidases. The use of this *in vitro* metabolic activation system has demonstrated that most known carcinogens (over 90 per cent) also possess mutagenic potential in *in vitro* test systems. Previously the correlation was poor but the possibility that *in vitro* mutagenic testing might also reveal carcinogenic potential has now become a matter of great importance. The last five years have seen an astonishing growth of knowledge in this area and already in the USA by February 1975 the 'Committee of 17' was able to publish its important summary of the situation.[5] It advocated that testing for mutagenesis was not only necessary but was a practical possibility. In the meantime the US Government's Department of Health Education and Welfare and the Environmental Protection Agency, the Canadian and Japanese Governments together with European Governments began to set up a variety of expert advisory bodies to produce guidelines on possible courses of action.

In the United Kingdom, the first official recognition of this was in 1970 when a small panel was set up to look into the implications of mutagenesis. This panel grew into a sub-committee and in January 1978 it became a full Standing Committee on the Mutagenicity of Chemicals in Food, Consumer Products and the Environment. Before considering how the UK Government is dealing with this very difficult problem some explanation of the Government machinery is necessary so that some aspects of the problem from the legislative and control point of view can be appreciated. Responsibility for the health of the nation is vested in the Department of Health and Social Security. This large Department has a Secretary of State and several ministers who are responsible to Parliament for its functions in all aspects of health, social security and pensions. On the health side the Chief Medical Officer is responsible for the advice given to ministers and others on professional aspects. He is assisted in this by a number of specialist divisions covering such subjects as hospital buildings, medical specialities and in the case of toxicology, the Division of Medical Aspects of Chemical Contamination of the Environment Food and Smoking. This is a Division, headed by a professional toxicologist, which has medical, scientific and administrative personnel and its job is to be aware of what is happening in all branches of toxicology and to provide advice in these fields to Central Government.

The Division is assisted in its work by a series of standing committees composed of experts in the appropriate subjects. The coordination of the widely diverse fields of importance in the assessment of possible environmental hazards and the work of the individual standing committees is the responsibility of a special committee chaired by the Chief Medical Officer. Each standing committee can be asked directly for scientific advice by other Government Departments or bodies such as the Ministry of Agriculture, Fisheries and Food and the Health and Safety Executive. Such scientific advice forms part of the risk/benefit analysis which precedes executive decisions by the responsible departments. The diverse interests in toxicology of Government Departments, Ministries and Statutory Authorities are coordinated by an Interdepartmental Committee. The activities of these two coordinating committees should ensure that all areas of concern in environmental health matters receive adequate and timely attention from the appropriate scientific advisers.

The DHSS Division of Medical Aspects of Chemical Contamination as part of its advisory function produces guidelines. For example it hopes early in 1979 to issue a consultative document on guidelines for mutagenicity testing. The question naturally arises as to the significance of such guidelines. The best parallel is the Highway Code which is not mandatory, that is, in law it has no absolute standing, but a proven breach of the Highway Code is in practice always taken into consideration in court proceedings concerning an alleged traffic offence. Thus the Mutagenicity Testing Guidelines, when finally agreed, will become the official scientific advice on this matter to Government Departments, Ministries and Statutory Authorities who have to implement the various pieces of legislation enacted by Parliament to protect the public from chemical hazards in their daily life, be it in their food, cosmetics, place of work or the general environment. There are for example a whole series of laws on the wholesomeness of foods. Thus the Ministries concerned with foods in the United Kingdom have ample powers to restrict or eliminate the use of a food additive if there is sufficient evidence to justify such action. Likewise the Health and Safety Executive have far reaching legislative powers to control the exposure of workers in their place of work to chemicals which are considered to be a hazard to health. It is the function of guidelines to provide the best scientific advice on the kind of evidence that is needed to establish that there is a hazard to health. It is the responsibility of the client departments to utilize this advice, together with any other advice relevant to the problem, to set out the toxicological testing requirements considered necessary to provide the scientific evidence needed for decision making.

Guidelines for toxicological or carcinogenesis testing have conformed in the past to a well understood pattern. Initially it was believed that a similar type of guideline would be possible for the detection of mutagens. Such a document was circulated by the Sub-Committee to industry for comment late in 1976. This was criticized mainly because the format chosen was believed to be unsuitable for a new subject in which knowledge was accumulating at an unprecedented rate. Thus an entirely new approach was needed. As mutagenesis was an entirely novel concept to many people and, as in its development it drew upon fundamental genetic knowledge which is also unfamiliar to even well informed biological scientists, it was decided that it might be helpful to have guidelines with a background of basic scientific concepts so that any proposals for mutagenicity testing could be viewed with some scientific perspective. It was therefore planned that the guidelines could consist of an introductory core document containing the rationale of why there was need for concern about genetic toxicology, and thus why there was a need for additional tests. This could be followed by sections dealing with the test proposals, what other test procedures were believed to be currently useful and how they might be best deployed, bearing in mind the limitations of any test procedure so far developed to detect mutagens.

It can be appreciated that the preparation of guidelines in this particular field poses many problems quite apart from the scientific issues which, as a number of speakers at this conference have indicated, are in many important practical matters still controversial. It would seem that whatever testing proposals are put forward must contain some element of compromise and flexibility. Such an approach is not easily accommodated by some legislative authorities where a rigid 'check-list' approach is favoured. The current proposals by the Environmental Protection Agency of the USA for the testing of pesticides, as set out recently in the Federal Register, have aroused much controversy because they follow this rigid line and the overall scheme if fully implemented in its present form for all chemicals would be prohibitively expensive. The DHSS's Committee on Mutagenesis has endeavoured to demonstrate that if the fundamental scientific principles of genetic toxicology are considered then a logical sequentual testing programme can be proposed which appears to have many advantages with little sacrifice of efficiency in the detection of possible hazard, bearing in mind the inherent uncertainties that are part of the current 'state of the art'.

A working paper along the above lines was presented for discussion at a meeting held under the auspices of the British Environmental Mutagen Society in November 1977. This was a most helpful meeting and following this and other informal discussions with colleagues from Europe and USA it is hoped that the Committee will finalise a consultative document early in 1979 which will set out proposals for a testing scheme. These proposals will be circulated for comment to Government Departments, Industrial Associations, appropriate academic bodies and any other bodies having responsibilities in the area. The Committee will then finalise their proposals in the light of the comments received and in due course a guideline document will be published.

There is an urgency to agree both nationally and internationally on a basic and realistic screening scheme for mutagenicity. Whatever system is devised has implications for capital investment in equipment and the training of people in the new technologies. At present the available facilities and skills are in no way commensurate with the number of chemicals proposed for testing. Thus any proposals by Government must be considered not only from the viewpoint of what they may or may not detect but also as to whether the scheme can be successfully carried out. Furthermore any test system should be capable of improvement without compromising the technologies which have been built up. Bearing in mind these constraints it can be argued, given the present state of knowledge, that the great majority of potentially hazardous chemicals can be detected by the systematic application of a combination of four test procedures which are designed to probe sequentially the hereditary machinery at increasing levels of complexity. Such a 'minimal package' of tests could be considered as a screening process for the detection of mutagens. Thus the first step is to detect mutagenic possibilities. The next step could be considered as the quite different process of the assessment of the significance of the findings regarding the hazard to man leading to the final process of risk/benefit analysis.

The 'minimum package' of tests could be based firstly on the bacterial auxotrophy to prototrophy reversion test systems (with and without metabolic activation) which is incontestably the most widely validated test system in the field of genetic toxicology; it is also believed to be the most sensitive. Although it must be recognized that this system will miss some mutagens, there is considerable evidence that when adequately used, that is with a suitable variety of lines and strains, mutagenic activity has been detected that was not apparent in the commonly used mammalian test systems. Few would disagree that a well conducted bacterial test for mutagenesis must constitute an essential part of any test scheme. A consequential proposition that further testing beyond the reversion system using micro-organisms should be directed at mammalian systems seems logical in a 'minimal package' concept.

A second test in the sequence follows from the fact that some genetic diseases result from demonstrable chromosome abnormalities and thus it would seem important to establish if a chemical possesses the ability to produce damage *in vitro* to chromosomes, as seen by optical microscopy at the metaphase stage of the mitotic cycle. This test procedure is particularly relevant because it need not be confined to cells from laboratory animals but can be carried out on human lymphocytes. Furthermore knowledge concerning cells including chromosomal damage is growing rapidly as are more sensitive methods for detecting it. The test can also be carried out with metabolic activation systems.

A third test procedure that can be suggested arises from the consideration that the bacterial genome is relatively simple compared to that of the mammalian cell and thus the path that a chemical must take to reach the chromatin and subsequently the DNA is quite different in prokaryotes and eukaryotes. Thus it seems logical to give high priority to a test concerned with gene mutation in mammalian cells in culture, using techniques based on the detection of mutagenesis at, for example, the loci for the hypoxanthine-guanine phosphoribosyl transferase or the thymidine kinase enzyme systems.

The tests so far discussed are based on *in vitro* techniques and thus have limitations although in both bacterial and tissue culture tests metabolic activation systems can be used to mimic *in vivo* metabolism. Thus logically an *in vivo* test should be included in the 'minimal package' to see how the chemical and its metabolites behave in the intact animal. Though different tests could be suggested it would seem that at present metaphase analysis of bone marrow in the rat or mouse is the most suitable.

A 'minimal package' of test procedures based on the above considerations if fully exploited should detect the potential mutagenic hazard of the great majority of chemicals. Opinions will differ but it could be as high as 95 % successful. Whatever the figure, it is quite clear that to improve on it at the screening level would entail an expenditure of effort out of all proportion to the value of the additional information that might be obtained. There is one notable omission in the suggested screen in that there is no proposed test for the detection of non-disjunction in mammals. At present there does not appear to be any validated test for this, yet it could be important in view of the frequency of numerical chromosome anomalies in man as causes of disease or reproductive casualty. It has also to be remembered that some non-disjunction could arise by mechanisms other than chemical interference.

From the regulatory point of view there is much to be said for starting on this new toxicological venture with a modest yet realistic set of proposals. There is a wide measure of agreement about the thirty or so test procedures that can produce acceptable evidence concerning the potential mutagenic hazard to man of a chemical. The debate is essentially about the deployment of the tests and the relevance of the results to man. If constraints in choice of tests must be applied then it is probably better to do this in the initial screening process which is designed to detect the hazard. By contrast in the next phase, that of evaluating the hazard to man, a more flexible approach is justified. Here as far as guidelines are concerned it is probably only useful to set out those 'supplementary tests' which the Committee judge to be acceptable internationally. Such a list could be added to as new knowledge appears. In addition it might be considered helpful to indicate what new scientific advances show promise of exploitation as a test system.

One advantage of a sequential approach to mutagen detection is that there may be circumstances where the use of a chemical will be limited and the degree of human exposure small or containable. In such situations a case could be made for accepting, as a first step, a 'mini package' of the first two suggested test procedures, that is, point mutations in bacteria and chromosomal damage *in vitro* in mammalian cells. Finally, if a 'minimal package' screening system proves to be acceptable and workable as a first step in this difficult and controversial area the state of knowledge is such that, because each test is directed at certain hereditary mechanisms, equivalent evidence derived from different systems could be accepted as alternatives to part of the package. However, the onus would have to be placed on the applicant to justify that the evidence produced was at least as good as would be expected from the tests suggested in the guidelines.

References

1. Gregg, N. M. (1941). Congenital cataract following German measles in the mother. *Trans. Ophthal. Soc. Aust.* **3,** 35
2. Deformities caused by Thalidomide. Report on Public Health and Medical Subjects. No 12, (1964). H.M. Stationary Office
3. Barnes, J. M. (1970). Aflatoxin as a health hazard. *Journal of Applied Bacteriology.* **33,** 285–298
4. Sugimura, T., Kawachi, T., Marsushima, J., Nagao, M., Sato, S. and Yahagi, T. (1977). A critical review of submammalian systems for mutagen detection. In Progress in Genetic Toxicology, Editors D. Scott, B. A. Bridges and F. H. Sobels. Elsevier, North-Holland Amsterdam, New York, Oxford. pp 125–140
5. Committee of 17, (1975). Environmental Mutagenic Hazards. *Science* **187,** 503–514

Discussion

Chairman: Dr G. E. Paget

Professor B. N. AMES (Berkeley): I agree with a number of the points that Dr Ashby raised and I disagree with a number of others. For example, he did not emphasize that animal cancer tests have their own problems, and as I pointed out in an earlier session, that became particularly clear in the case of the Japanese food additive where there were not only one, but two, negative cancer tests, and then it came out positive in a whole series of short-term tests, and the people went back and re-did the animal cancer tests more thoroughly and it turned out that it was a carcinogen. So I am not quite convinced that some of the false positives Dr Ashby raised are really false positives. I think in a number of those cases one should really look more thoroughly at the animal cancer tests, although there are certainly some false negatives.

One powerful tool is a battery of short-term tests, like the fact that some of the short-term tests can be optimized and each one is still being improved. Then we shall have this battery, and then the mistake level will go down drastically. I think it still remains to be seen how many false positives there are. The false negatives will become fewer as we learn of what each substance is doing. Clearly there will be a class of substances that do not work directly on the DNA, but in some indirect way, and we shall need systems for that.

Dr B. J. DEAN (Sittingbourne): Professor Ames mentioned batteries of tests, and I should like to say one word about the use of batteries. The present consensus is not to use just the one or two tests, but a battery. The short-term tests that have been published over the last 2 years, including things like microbial tests, yeast, transformation assays, chromosomal exchanges, DNA repair, chromosome assays– invariably use, as a method – as a metabolizing system – an S-9 mix. If the balance in the S-9 is not right for that particular compound, then they will all be negative, and no matter how many tests are included in the battery, there will be a negative result.

Dr Ashby has made the point very clearly to ring the changes with the metabolizing system as well as with the end point. He has also made out a very good case for the development of *in vivo* assays, short term *in vivo* assays. There are so many problems involved with mimicking mammalian metabolism, physiology, etc. *in vitro* that I feel that during the next few years the next forward step in this direction must be development of short-term assays using the whole animal.

Dr PAGET (Inveresk): We owe a debt to Dr Ashby for a most stimulating paper, and I should like to pay a compliment to the ICI group. It is wholly laudable to see an industrial laboratory establish this outstanding team in this advancing area, and thus contributing very significantly to our knowledge. I would couple with that Dr Dean's Group at Shell. Both these groups are greatly to be complimented.

Dr J. ASHBY (Macclesfield): I have two brief points that back up Dr Oftedal's discussion.

First, in *Mutation Research* (Vol 54) in the very last brief communication, there is a discussion of folpet, captan, and related compounds, where the problem is approached of how they are positive *in vitro* and yet apparently non-carcinogenic. Some very interesting experiments were done which relate to the Class 2 false positives that I discussed earlier. One can get a *Salmonella* positive with these compounds that is immediately abolished when blood is added to the assay medium, or when serum is added, and eventually it was tied right down to cysteine levels, and it was the SH Group on cysteine which was abolishing the effect of active species – so that relates to Class 2 false positives.

That is one way. The other way is the amytrol data. There are two relevant pieces of information. One is that it is to aminotriazol, which happens to be positive, it was mentioned earlier, in cell transformation – which is another interesting aspect of two systems looking at the same compound. I believe there is now data to the affect that although it is a thyroid carcinogen that could simply be associated with the hormonal function, it actually induces malignant effects in the associated areas. So it looks as if that may be a carcinogen, albeit weak, but a genuine one, and perhaps Norway's stand is not too bad.

Professor B. N. AMES: I hate to discuss Captan. This is getting off the general subject – but

The first cancer tests that were done on Captan, they dissolved it in a protein solution, and one might expect that the Captan might have reacted with the protein. It may be that Captan does react very quickly with thiol groups – but maybe if people are breathing in the Captan dust, it may be that it will cause lung cancer even though it would not if it were fed. So we still have to treat it with respect and to worry whether Captan is really a non-carcinogen, to see what the route of exposure is, and to think about that as well. We may want to try animal experiments in a similar route of exposure to the one that people are getting.

Dr Diana ANDERSON (Macclesfield): Dr Draper says that the Guidelines are to be published in the autumn (1978) and that he will then expect comments from industry. What are the nature of the comments that are expected this time?

Dr M. H. DRAPER (London): This is a formal process that must be gone through by any guideline document. It may be that if industry likes the document, they will not make any comments. This is rather unlikely. But I think that industry, or those concerned in industry, could write back. They could agree with it, or they could disagree with it. They could suggest ways it might be improved. This is a process that we are obliged to go through, and that is only right.

Because of our previous contact with industry, we hope we have in a sense met a great deal of the objections that industry had had previously, but of course when industry has sent in comment we must digest the whole lot, and then we have to agree. The Committee has to recommend a final document which then goes to the chief medical office, to the Minister of State, and it then becomes, if agreed, the equivalent of a White Paper.

In a sense, once that document is out in consultative form, and once it has come back, then industry will know that what we intend to suggest is the necessity for bacteriological technology and for tissue technology. How these technologies are deployed may change, but the two technologies are with us for at least the next decade. Industry are pretty clear about this.

In effect industry will be able to choose *S. typhimurium* or *E. coli*. If any part of industry chooses to come up with a test that is well validated, the

Committee would certainly accept it if it was scientific – a dominant lethal from the rat for example – but at the moment I think one could go a long way on the somatic side in a screen. There are germ-cell tests coming along which in a year one might be able to suggest are taken on board, but efficient culture technology will still be needed. But if we should get into attacking the germ cell directly, we would then be into fairly big experiments, and we feel we should start very gently.

Professor B. N. AMES: I have one point on bacterial systems versus mammalian systems. In a way, the *Salmonella* test is ground-up rat liver or ground-up human liver plus bacteria, and the bacteria would be used to measure damage to DNA. If one looks at unscheduled DNA synthesis and one uses ground-up liver plus an animal cell for measuring unscheduled DNA synthesis, one would really be using the same ground-up rat liver as one models for mammalian metabolism in two different ways of looking at DNA damage. So in a way all these systems are mixed systems, and one has to ask what one can get out of them. In some cases using primary liver cells – should someone develop a system like that – they are directly activating material and the ground-up liver will not be needed. But then maybe the human liver cannot be used in that system. So each of them has various aspects, but in some sense they are all combined mammalian systems.

Dr DRAPER: I accept that, with the provision that where one is doing metaphase analysis, particularly *in vivo*, the tissue culture technology will still be needed to look at the metaphase analysis. But I take the point.

But I think we get a little bit extra out of the mammalian cells.

Professor AMES: I think there should be a battery of systems.

Dr DRAPER: We have a primitive little 1.5 volt battery here.

Dr R. S. MANN (Guildford): I thought I heard Dr Draper say that he wanted to make sure that when the findings were negative, they were as significant as any other findings. What does that mean? In the presence of a negative finding or no difference, I can understand being puzzled about a beta error, but not an alpha error. What do we mean by making a negative finding significant?

Dr DRAPER: It merely means establishing biological variability in the control. In effect it is establishing the null hypothesis – one would always test the null hypothesis. Therefore one can say that the result is negative, and that the chance of its being a false negative – it could be 1/20 or 1/100 by chance – that one could be missing a positive result.

Perhaps I can refer Dr Mann to Professor Ehrenberg's Paper on the null hypothesis.

Dr A. MUNN (Brussels): Dr Draper referred to the importance of disasters in stimulating part of our problems, but one disaster to which he did not refer, perhaps the most publicized disaster in recent years where there has been massive public exposure to chemical mutagenic agents, has been the Seveso affair. We all remember the prophecies of doom and gloom at the time, and we know some of the subsequent events. We know that there was a fair number of people who suffered from alkali burns, that there were a limited, and surprisingly small number of cases of chloroacne. What about evidence of mutagenic effect in people who were exposed? We know that there were many surgical terminations of pregnancy immediately after Seveso, and it has been suggested that this may have been the most disastrous aspect of all. However, in babies conceived in the period immediately before Seveso, and subsequently born, has there been evidence of genetic defects? In babies conceived of parents in the area of Seveso, but conceived after the disaster, has there been evidence of genetic defects? Have there been chromosome studies of the people involved, and if so what have been the results of these chromosome studies?

Dr DRAPER: A certain amount of this work has been done, but I gather from the reports that we have that there have been certain difficulties in getting at the people. The results so far, in terms of the disaster, have been, as Dr Munn suggests, surprisingly small. But one must not forget that some of the troubles that might beset us, which were mentioned by Professor Bridges, may not appear until the people are 30 or 40 years old – Huntington's chorea for example. We still have to reserve judgment. I do not think that the full Seveso findings are yet available. There is a considerable amount of worry about the litigation possibilities, which does tend to make life difficult.

What information we have is that the results are surprisingly negative. As Dr Munn suggests, the abortion side appeared to be all right, but we do not know whether chromosomal studies were carried out on the abortuses. We just do not know.

ROUND TABLE DISCUSSION
Chairman: Lord Ritchie-Calder

WRITTEN QUESTION: What do the experts recommend in respect of monitoring for the mutagenic effects of chemicals on reproductive function? Is the three-generation mouse study considered adequate in this respect? Is there any simpler/quicker method available?

Professor AMES: I was quite impressed by the assay that Bruce and Warbeck published on sperm abnormalities in mice. In mouse sperm, the tail of the sperm is apparently determined by many hundreds of genes, and there is a certain low rate of sperm abnormalities which can be determined by looking – by pointing out a few thousand sperm on a slide and looking at them. The authors of the study fed all kinds of chemicals to the mice and irradiated them, and they could see a dose-response relation in increase in sperm abnormalities for a high percentage of the carcinogens fed. I thought it quite an interesting paper, and it might be a simple way of looking at that kind of question – at what chemicals are actually getting to the germ line. It may be slightly different from the standard reproductive test.

Dr ANDERSON: That assay is more a somatic assay of germ cells, just looking at the morphological changes. The questioner was after transmissible genetic damage. If we want to look at progressive damage transmitted through several generations, then with the kind of study suggested, abnormal offspring can be eaten by the mother, and a false picture of what is really happening might result. A heritable translocation study, measuring the F_1 generation effects on litter size, will give an idea of transmissible damage. It can be got from the other study, but that might give a false picture.

Dr DEAN: One point on sperm abnormality. There are one or two peculiar things about it. For example, by increasing the temperature of the mouse testes one can get a temperature-related increase in sperm abnormalities per degree Centigrade. So there are one or two peculiar factors that influence sperm abnormalities. There are also strain differences. There are strains of mice where it is possible to get something like 90–95 % of the sperm with abnormal tails.

Professor AMES: I am not sure that that is the reason. Heat is mutagenic, and the reason why men wear kilts or have their testicles outside of their bodies may be to keep them cool. Because heat gives an increase in sperm abnormalities, it does not mean that it is a bad assay. In the particular strain they were looking at there is a fairly low rate. They have even looked at people, but there are so many sperm abnormalities in males that it is hard to do. But I think that someone has now shown that cigarette smoke gives some increase in sperm abnormality.

I think Warbeck and Bruce have done some studies showing that these are passed on to the next generation.

Dr DEAN: Yes, that is true. And they have also done a correlation between sperm abnormalities and translocations.

Mr N. J. Van ABBE (Leatherhead, Surrey): I would suggest that the validity of the mutagenicity findings is at risk of being under-rated through making comparisons against an all-or-none classification of 'carcinogens' and 'non-carcinogens'. Would it not be more helpful to re-classify suspect compounds according to whether or not they show potent mutagenic activity? For example, should compounds producing only injection-site sarcomas be regarded as 'carcinogens' when considering their behaviour in mutagenicity tests?

Dr ASHBY: I am sure that Professor Ames will come back to the initial part of the question, and I will support what he says.

On the last point, with a subcutaneous injection experiment of whose significance I was unsure, because it is known that there is a spontaneous rate through sticking in the needle, then I would suggest that, if there are two compounds both producing local tumours at the site of subcutaneous injection, then if one is positive *in vitro* and the other is negative, I would pay much more attention to the positive and assume that with a full study it would be a general carcinogen. I would also – but this reflects my own interest – superimpose on that whether or not it made sense chemically that one or the other of them was reactive and producing cancer.

Professor AMES: I pass.

Mr Van ABBE: For example, in listing carcinogens and non-carcinogens when tabulating mutagens, would those substances which only produce a subcutaneous sarcoma be included as carcinogens?

Dr STYLES: In the ICI study, these were not considered to be carcinogens – but it is a debatable point.

Dr ASHBY: And there were not many of them, so they do not have much influence on the overall figures. One or two at the most.

Mr Van ABBE: To come back again. What about the compounds that only produce hepatomas in mice?

Dr ASHBY: They, likewise, were excluded in that study. In particular, DDT and dieldrin were considered non-carcinogens, and the short-term tests were scored up because they found them negative. But that is another topic.

Dr DEAN: I think it is a mechanism of carcinogenicity that the short-term tests in their present form will not detect the process where one has liver cell hyperplasia, hyperplastic modules, which then go on to produce – to change into carcinomas. This appears to be a different mechanism of carcinogenesis.

Professor AMES: We called those false negatives carcinogens and said that the *Salmonella* test was not picking up many of them, and we shall just have to see how it comes out.

Dr ASHBY: That comes full circle. In a way you are scoring your test down and if there is another mechanism you come right back to the question, you are discrediting the test, when it perhaps necessarily is not true.

Professor EHRENBERG: This is an interesting question because it refers to the various classifications which have been done as something *either/or*, according to some kind of all or none consideration.

Take a compound like ethylene, or ethane, the simplest of the alkanes. We tried it with the so-called Ames test and it was negative, but we could see alkylation of proteins and DNA *in vivo* of animals. Probably no cancer test has been done with this compound and it is generally considered to be non-carcinogenic and non-mutagenic. In the industrial lists of toxicity, the limit set is asphyxiation – when such a high concentration is reached that there is the risk of lack of oxygen, or the risk of explosion – the explosion danger. But if we accept the reality of dose–response curves, the compound is certainly a false negative in the mutation tests, and it would become a false negative in any cancer test. A risk is certainly involved – which is the order of magnitude comparable to the risk from background radiation – when we consider the level of ethylene in urban air.

According to my philosophy we do not want to use the words 'non-carcinogens' and 'non-mutagens' unless we have considerable chemical proof that the compounds cannot react with DNA, or that they cannot, through metabolism or some other action, give rise to chemicals which can react with DNA. In that event they could be called non-carcinogens and non-mutagens. In any case, a negative test should always be provided with the confidence interval so that when a compound is judged non-mutagenic or non-carcinogenic what is meant is less than a certain frequency which is up to the 95% confidence interval, or something like that.

In addition to the false positives and false negatives that Dr Ashby discussed, there are the false positives and the false negatives that are false for statistical reasons.

Mr N. J. Van ABBE: Professor Ames referred to substances enhancing mutagenicity without themselves being mutagenic. Are these enhancers related to those known to act as co-carcinogens in animal studies? Is it possible to show in mutagenicity tests whether the enhancer and the mutagen interact to give enhanced effect when administered separately?

Professor AMES: Many interesting cases are now being turned up where two chemicals are synergistic in the mutagenicity assay, or they interfere with each other, and it would be very interesting to work out how they behave when they are used in animal cancer tests. Dr Ashby talked about it, and Sugamura has done a lot of work – the Norharman plus aniline, and so on. One can imagine many reasons for that – as Dr Ashby pointed out – inhibiting some pathway that normally takes the chemical down some harmless path, and that then converts it to a mutagen. We are working on an idea that for certain mutagens, there might be an inter-colating agent that unwinds the DNA a bit and produces some single stranded region, and then the mutagen can hit that. One can think of several examples, both metabolic, and such as I have just described, where there might be interaction between chemicals, and then there is a whole class of promotors in all of that. Hopefully the short-term tests will help to sort it out and one can then double-check it with animal cancer tests.

Dr ASHBY: One word of caution about synergism experiments. I am sure there will be several mechanisms by which synergism can be produced, and I am sure that in some circumstances the explanation I put up this morning will hold. There will be other explanations and I am not sure which one Norharman is in.

But, a word of caution on extrapolating it to *in vivo*. We have noticed in the *in vivo/in vitro* experiments that you get no effect – the experiments I showed were just doubling the dose. For example; one of azobenzene, one of Butter Yellow. Initially there is no effect, then suddenly, at a given dose of azobenzene the effect starts, and there is a wide divergence in the Butter Yellow, or the Butter Yellow plus azobenzene. This seems consistent with a coligative theory of enzyme competition – that it needs a certain dose. In the extreme, an azobenzene will be needed on every enzyme surface of the azoreductase before the Butter Yellow is rescued, and the dose of azobenzene to do that in terms of the *in vitro* test is very high. If that is extrapolated to man, there would have to be a very high level of azobenzene in his liver before any low levels of Butter Yellow would have an extraordinary effect.

One has to bear in mind that one may be absolutely blocking an enzyme and that may take a lot of material, which does not look very much in an *in vitro* test on the S-9 but may be a great amount *in vivo*, and that if a man is exposed to azobenzene and Butter Yellow, the azobenzene will not significantly affect the azoreductase system and the Butter Yellow will be just as bad, or as good, as it was initially.

Dr J. WIERIKS (Delft, The Netherlands): Is there an increase in frequency of inherited genetic diseases, either in number, or in 'new' diseases? If not, would it mean that that type of genetic disease is multigenetically determined, so that more mutations are necessary?

On the other hand, the frequency of cancer has apparently increased under the influence of environmental carcinogenesis. Would the conclusion be that it is easier to develop cancer than genetic inheritable diseases?

Professor AMES: Professor Bridges pointed out that it is really very hard to monitor human genetic defects, and that the epidemiology is very unsatisfactory on this. I do not think that anybody really knows how much of that is caused by environmental agents. It would be nice to have more efficient monitoring systems for that in case the genetic effects suddenly started to double, but one may find many slight effects that are hard to pin down.

As for the cancer rate going up, the experts agree that it is not really going up except for cigarette smoking, and that mostly the rate is pretty constant. That has been one of the arguments, that a lot of the cancer today may well be dietary; that is, that it may be in our normal exposure. So apart from ultra-violet light and cigarette smoking there is not that much of an increase in general cancer rates. In my own presentation I coupled that with the point that we would not expect to see too much from the modern chemical world until the 1980 decade, so that can be thrown in for whatever it is worth.

Dr ANDERSON: One of the difficulties with monitoring genetic damage is that some of the end points are recessive in nature and will not show for many generations. We could go along for many years before we picked them up. I go along with all the points that Professor Ames made.

Dr DEAN: Just a minor point. During the last 30 or 40 years there has been an apparent increase in genetic types of diseases. This is really because over that period clinicians have only really recognized those diseases as having some genetic association, and I think that people are still recognizing particular syndromes as having some genetic input. Until we reach a stage where much more is known about genetic disease, where much more is found about the genetic association of such conditions as diabetes, for example, where there is a great deal of doubt about the genetic association, we have no baseline from which to measure.

Dr OFTEDAL: Regarding genetic disease, in man there are really only two materials that give us proper numbers. In the mid-fifties, Stevenson investigated the population of Northern Ireland. He saw practically every malformed child that was born there over a period and pinned down the various conditions to their genetic categories to the extent that they were known or thought to be genetically determined. Stevenson arrived at a number for dominantly inherited genetic disease, 1%, which was used by the United Nations Committee in 1958. Then some 15 years later, in Canada, Howard Newcome and his pupil Ben Thrimble, collected numbers and data from British Columbia on the basis of a different type of survey, from registries, social insurance, etc. where a much larger population could be monitored. They arrived at a figure of 0.1% – a factor of 10 down relative to Stevenson's estimate. Those are the only two figures that we have.

I happen to chair a small task group within the Radiological Protection

Commission. Dr Thrimble was one of our members and another was Professor Cedric Carter of London who has clinical experience. We also had Friedrich Folgen, who also has clinical experience in man. After they had discussed Thrimble's data, and also the Thrimble and Doughty data from British Columbia, that figure of dominantly inherited disease was again raised to 1 %, but it was a different 1 % from the one that Stevenson had presented.

This is the level of our Foundation now; that a single man, or a small group of experts is able to twist this number by a factor of 10 up and down.

The UNSKA Committee also uses 1 %, and that is probably because Cedric Carter was a member of the British delegation.

With regard to cancer frequency, I think there is – or there used to be – a steady increase in Scandinavia in leukaemia, since the 1940s or so, it has been going up by a few per cent per year. But this was thought to be almost entirely a diagnostic increase.

On the other hand, apart from lung cancer, there is a real increase over the last 15 years in malignant melanomas. These are associated with the areas of the skin that are exposed to sunlight, and they are increasing in Norway because people can now take cheap charter flights to the Majorcas and to the Canary Islands. It is a question of what price people pay for the added health of sunning themselves, and swimming in winter, having 14 hours of sunlight instead of 3 hours per day.

Dr J. WIERIKS: The problem of the no-carcinogenic effect level still exists. Could we get indications for the existence of such a level from no-muta-genic-effect levels, e.g. in bacterial tests?

Dr DEAN: No. I believe it is a problem of thresholds, and we all have our own views and could talk about it for several hours. I am prepared to leave it at that. I hold the view that in certain instances there could be a threshold. Professor Ames might have a different view – that there is no such thing as a threshold.

Professor AMES: I would not be surprised if certain chemicals did have a threshold. On the other hand, I suspect that most do not, but they may not all be the same. We do not know.

Dr ANDERSON: I suspect that some do. Radiation and radiomimetic chemicals like alkylating agents might not have thresholds, but there are so many chemicals in industry which do not behave in this way that I would be very surprised if they did not have thresholds.

Dr DEAN: There is a little experimental evidence for thresholds. For example, there are one or two compounds that we have tested in the microbial system with the conventional S-9 fractions where we can show a mutagenic activity. If we then add to the system physiological concentrations of, for example, glutathione, we eliminate the mutagenic activity completely in the bacterial system. Whether this means that *in vivo* the glutathione will mop up that compound up to a certain concentration, and then as soon as the cysteine or the glutathione or whatever is saturated there will be an effect *in vivo*, I do not know, and it has never been shown. It is one possible theory of thresholds.

Professor AMES: Maybe we should not get on to thresholds, but the case that Dr Ashby mentioned might be a good theoretical example of a way of getting thresholds. It takes a certain level to inhibit a particular pathway. The alkylating agent – glutathione and DNA are competing and there is always some fraction that is hitting the DNA. Whether that would give you a threshold or not I do not know, unless the glutathione was finally saturated.

Professor EHRENBERG: To add to what Dr Dean said. If we consider risk in man, I do not believe that we could define a certain concentration as *the* physiological concentration of glutathione. It could be that with an inbred animal strain, there is a very narrow variation around a certain mean value. But in man there are enormous variations in such respects, both within a population and between populations. This means a variation in risk with regard to such an effect as is being discussed.

Take the mercury catastrophe in Iraq a few years ago. The concentrations were quite tolerable by European populations, but because those concerned lacked glutathione, they were much more sensitive.

Dr J WIERIKS: If for cancer-induction concentration times exposure time is necessary, could that lead to the conclusion that some mutagenicity (carcinogenicity) is acceptable for drugs which are used only during very short periods of human life?

Professor EHRENBERG: This concerns a problem which was touched upon in one of the sessions. The importance of not discussing a simple Yes or No was pointed out. In situations where there is real benefit from a certain chemical, it must be discussed in terms of How and To What Extent.

It is quite true that certain chemicals could be given at high concentrations if applied for a short time. Since risk is proportional to dose, if dose is concentration times time, the risk would be so small that the treatment or the exposure would be acceptable even if given to young people who may be prospective parents.

It touches on a general point, namely, there are many chemicals in industry that are of such an economic value, or value to human health or wellbeing in other respects, that these chemicals have to be lived with in some way even though they have been shown to be mutagenic and carcinogenic. It is an extremely difficult situation for the administrators, to suggest something which could lead to tragedies, to cancers, to malformed children. Yet we do it with radiation at present.

Professor AMES: I would agree with Professor Ehrenberg. It is not a question of if something is a mutagen then ban it, because there are many carcinogens that people are using all the time that have not been banned, and everyone agrees. There are even carcinogens in people, like vinyl chloride. Before it was known to be a carcinogen it was used in millions of spray cans, and women were breathing in 300 ppm in the bathroom, and workers were breathing in 200 ppm or whatever. We want to know that, and to treat it with respect, but there is still an enormous vinyl plastics industry and we have not shut it down.

All of this information should go into regulatory agencies and they can then take it all into consideration. Practically all the anti-cancer drugs are carcinogens, yet they are still useful as anti-cancer drugs. A particular drug might be useful for curing a specific condition, one takes it once and one is finished. All these questions will have to be addressed. We shall not ban all carcinogens. There will be many useful chemicals that we shall know are carcinogens, but we shall want to know what their hazards are, as best we can, and treat them with respect.

Dr ANDERSON: It might be worth going a little further with the vinyl chloride story. It has certainly not been banned, but it has been treated with great respect. Within our own industry, for example, levels have been considerably reduced, and on the workshop there are points throughout the workshop where the concentrations are monitored constantly. These points are analyzed and thrown out on a computer, and the analyses are available for the men to see, and to monitor levels. In fact there are very strict controls. So it seems that we can live with known hazards if they are looked at sensibly.

Professor AMES: The regulatory agencies may even want to take short-term test information seriously. I was heavily involved with the TRIS story in the US. Fifteen million children were exposed to a chemical that was added to polyester as a flame retardant, with minimum toxicology before this enormous experiment was started. Five per cent, or ten per cent of the weight of the pyjama was this flame retardant, over an enormous surface area, of millions of children. Just looking at the chemical it looked dangerous, with all those bromines on it. It came up as a mutagen in *Salmonella*, and it was also quickly found to be a mutagen in *Drosophila*, and chromosomal exchange and mouse lymphoma, and yet even with all that it was a long time before the animal cancer tests came out and we could not even get the regulatory agency to label the garments that had TRIS. Some of the environmental groups were pushing the regulatory agency just to put a label on it that it contained TRIS, not even to ban it, just on the basis of all this mutagenicity, and yet we could not even get them to do that. Perhaps short-term tests should also be taken into consideration. In this case polyester was relatively flame-resistant and the whole story was perhaps silly in the first place.

All this toxicological information has to be considered, and a decision may be made on many types of information.

Dr DRAPER: Professor Ames is absolutely right, and so is Dr Anderson. We shall have to learn about these chemicals, and some of them we shall have to live with. The basic thing is to understand as much as we can about the possibilities of the molecules acting on human DNA. We may have to extrapolate from animals, but we have to take what people call 'the toxicological profile'. There are many other aspects of toxicology, apart from these, and then we have to do this very difficult risk–benefit estimation. This will be a matter for the various regulatory agencies – to get all the possible information they can. The decision making will be extremely difficult, and at the moment we do not have the data base to proceed very far. The case of TRIS is very revealing. It is very hard to push against the very big vested commercial interests. But each case like TRIS makes it a little easier for the next – we hope.

Professor AMES: To speak up for industry. The problem with TRIS was the Government. There is a lot of blame to share around, but it was a government commission – the Consumer Products Safety Commission – that was established to do something about children catching fire, and it made these very strict rules about flammability of fabrics, so that an industry – at least the sleepwear industry – that did not want to do this had to meet those standards. Then the company that made the chemical did not worry too much about the toxicology and all the sleepwear manufacturers were caught in the middle. It was a very complicated case. Sometimes governments can be at fault in these cases.

Dr J WIERIKS: Some day some one will find some new drug, say a curariform substance, which would only be used during anaesthesia, which is once or twice in a lifetime. In all the modern tests it proves to be

mutagenic or carcinogenic, and I fear we shall have great difficulty convincing the authorities that it is worthwhile putting it on the market. There
are already so many good drugs, why take the risk? Everybody knows
that as yet there is no ideal curariform agent.

Or to take another example, a new antibiotic which would be used now
and then in pneumonia, for 5 days. How many people get pneumonia?

This is the point. Something is found which is of great value, and it is
found to have a measure of mutagenicity or carcinogenicity, than we in the
pharmaceutical industry will say that we should forget about it, we do not
want difficulties with the authorities. If they start to say No, we shall have
to convince them, it will be very time-consuming, and we cannot afford
that loss of time.

Dr DRAPER: The situation with drugs is rather simpler because there are
occasions where there is a clear benefit, an established benefit. On the
particular example of a curariform drug people have speculated that
these are specific receptor sites. They attach specifically – not co-valent
bonding – and therefore they are very unlikely, by the nature of their
interaction, to interact with DNA. That has been a speculation.

For schistosomiasis we are already accepting that the benefits greatly
outweigh the risks, and we know that we are dealing with a dangerous
compound.

In the case of medicines, certainly in Britain, the Committee for Safety
of medicines would evaluate the risk – benefit very carefully. In any case,
for drugs there is far more information than for any other substance. There
is a whole toxicological profile, and a fairly balanced judgment can be
made.

It is not as gloomy – at least in Britain it is not as gloomy on the drug
side as it might be on the chemical side. We have far more information, and
we can get a very good idea of the benefits – which is the important thing.

All medicines are poisons. Every time one prescribes for a patient one
weighs up whether it is better that he has the drug than that he does not
have it – or one should.

Mr R GRIGGS (Haslemere, Surrey): How do the various tests cope with
the problem of endogenous or dietary mutagens, e.g. some of the aromatic
components of Allium. What is the relevance of positive results to human
risk and the implications of the results from structural analogues?

Professor AMES: I think it is becoming clear that there are a lot of
mutagens in normal diet. That point was made several times. Plants have
been devising nasty chemicals to kill off the insects that have been chewing

them for many million years. Nature is not benign, and all kinds of natural products are turning up that are mutagens and may well be carcinogens. Some of them people may have learned to handle in evolution, or to handle them reasonably well, others maybe not, and the public will soon get fed up with being told that mustard is mutagenic or onion is mutagenic. There will be a lot of mutagens out there and that is just the way it will turn out. Nobody yet knows what the risk is, or how much we have learnt to handle these substances. There may even be racial differences in how people have learned to handle them in evolution, and so it gets complicated.

Dr Emil POULSEN (Denmark): I am on the regulatory side, but I am perhaps being unfair to the Panel in posing a question which has been in the air in my own country. It is a question of benefit. Who is to judge benefit for others. In Denmark, some workers were told by a group working with the Ames test that the epoxy resins were mutagenic and probably carcinogenic, and they said that they would not work with these substances, and they went on strike. They accepted the argument that these substances might not be carcinogenic in the end, and they accepted that the substances should be tested in long-term tests, and some were tested and were found to be suspected carcinogens – that is another matter. What the workers said was that they did not wish to be the guinea pigs. They had no objection to the scientists finding out in 5 years time whether or not the substances were carcinogens, but they had no wish to be exposed to them in the meantime, because they did not see that they had any personal benefit from their use. Of course society may benefit. Those who have the job done may benefit. But does the worker have any benefit? Where does he come in the considerations? And who is to judge such benefit?

I was fortunate in that it did not end up in my regulatory area.

Dr DRAPER: It is a very difficult area.

In the UK there is a specific organization to consider the problem of the safety of the worker at his work – the Health and Safety Executive (HSE), in which the trades unions play an active part. It may be the way to solve that question. There will be many instances where workers might choose to ask such a question, but they may not always choose to give the answer that that particular group in Denmark gave. But we have to face up to the question.

In the UK, we have a body whose specific job it is to look at that very point, and if it is not safe for the workers to work in these conditions, then something would have to be done about it. They would have to decide what is to be done. It might be that a solution could be found by containment or something of that sort, but that must be the way to go. We cannot dodge that one. We have to face up to it.

Professor EHRENBERG: Dr Poulson has raised an important question – that those who benefit are not those who run the risk. In the long run, when the calculations are done, those who strike in that situation themselves benefit from other activities where others take the risk. It has to be dealt with on a larger scale. The workmen could be given the right to refuse to work with epoxy resins on condition that they do not expose the public to carcinogenic fumes from their car exhausts – that they do not use their cars, or are responsible for the special risks to gasolenc station workers who must deal with the fumes from the gasolene. There is a whole ream of such situations in society which have to be discussed.

Professor AMES: Unions and workers will have to become more knowledgeable about a lot of these areas. I have been surprised at how little chemical workers' unions have been concerned about chemicals and it seems to me that there will have to be a lot of arguing back and forth between unions and chemical companies, in addition to the government getting involved. The people who are concerned should know what the risks are, and yet in general, at least in the US, workers do not know what chemicals they are working with. The DBCP workers did not know that they were handling a carcinogen. So the more information around, the better. One of the roles of government is to provide information.

   People are willing to smoke cigarettes where there is an enormous risk – 10 years of his life for the two-pack-a-day smoker – and it does not seem to bother them. So there are risks in the world, but as far as possible governments should be involved in saying what information we have and letting people work it out – knowing what the risks are and letting people take it from there.

Mr N. J. Van ABBE: I nearly had a strike on my hands in my own (Beechams) Laboratories when it came to finding a volatile positive control for mutagenicity testing. Would any member of the Panel like to make suggestions for a reasonably safe volatile positive control?

Dr DEAN: By its very nature there is no such thing. If one wants to use volatile positive controls in a laboratory, then one has to design the laboratory to handle them safely so that none of the staff can conceivable be exposed to them. Laboratory designing is heading that way now, so that this can be done.

   I do not blame the Beechams staff at all.

ROUND TABLE DISCUSSION-
CONCLUDING REMARKS
Lord Ritchie-Calder

Dr Paget has done me a greater service than I appreciated in the first instance. I had thought I was coming to be informed about the advances – which I have been – and the techniques and so forth. But in this Round Table discussion I have found myself involved in another way. In my other incarnation I happen to be a parliamentarian – as a member of the House of Lords – and I sympathize so much with Dr Draper, and with Dr Oftedal, in the problems of coping with the necessity of regulation. It is a real problem. We have listened to the arguments on both sides, and the trouble with scientists is that they see both sides. There was that famous remarks of Senator Muskie in a Senate Inquiry in the US when the scientists in succession were coming up and saying: 'On the one hand this, and on the other hand that', and Muskie said: 'For God's sake send us a one-armed scientist.' It is difficult to make up one's mind.

What we were discussing when we were trying to define levels and so on were regulatory practices. We were talking about the philosophy of risk. The philosophy of risk, whether it be maximum permissible dosage of radiation or whatever it may be, is the philosophy of risk. Legislation for road transport sets speed limits for particular roads, and such limits have no relevance to the speed of the car, or to what it is capable of. What we are doing is to lay down the definition within which we expect people to behave, including scientists, industry and so forth – to behave within limits which will not add additional risk. Yet most of the time, as we saw from these discussions, every time somebody got up, they were exposing a new kind of risk. We have this mounting information on hazards, we must come to terms with it, and the main point is, as Professor Ames said, that it is an education question – and one that extends to the House of Lords and to Members of Parliament, because that is where the decisions will ultimately rest, in the definition of our responsibility to the general public.

I have found this a very illuminating conference, and I am sure that everybody who participated, from whatever aspect he looked at it, has obtained a great deal of insight and information, and probably new ideas. I certainly did.

Index

225